Stay Amazing Em

love

Barbara

x

LAND OF THE RISING LIFESPAN

Japanese Rituals of Longevity

Barbara Lovesy

BALBOA.PRESS

A DIVISION OF HAY HOUSE

Balboa Press books may be ordered through booksellers or by contacting:

Balboa Press
A Division of Hay House
1663 Liberty Drive
Bloomington, IN 47403
www.balboapress.co.uk
UK TFN: 0800 0148647 (Toll Free inside the UK)
UK Local: (02) 0369 56325 (+44 20 3695 6325 from outside the UK)

Because of the dynamic nature of the Internet, any web addresses or links contained in this book may have changed since publication and may no longer be valid. The views expressed in this work are solely those of the author and do not necessarily reflect the views of the publisher, and the publisher hereby disclaims any responsibility for them.

The author of this book does not dispense medical advice or prescribe the use of any technique as a form of treatment for physical, emotional, or medical problems without the advice of a physician, either directly or indirectly. The intent of the author is only to offer information of a general nature to help you in your quest for emotional and spiritual well-being. In the event you use any of the information in this book for yourself, which is your constitutional right, the author and the publisher assume no responsibility for your actions.

Any people depicted in stock imagery provided by Getty Images are models, and such images are being used for illustrative purposes only. Certain stock imagery © Getty Images.

Interior Image Credit: Paul Saberton

Print information available on the last page.

ISBN: 979-8-7652-1561-6 (sc)
ISBN: 979-8-7652-1560-9 (hc)
ISBN: 979-8-7652-1559-3 (e)

Library of Congress Control Number: 2025918045

Balboa Press rev. date: 08/27/2025

Contents

Introduction

Konichiwa, I'm Barbara, and I'm so thrilled that you've decided to explore this book with me. Japan has truly captured my heart and soul, and after living there for 10 years, it has become an integral part of who I am.

The wisdom, tranquility, and deeply rooted wellness traditions of Japan continue to influence my life today, and I am excited to share some of these practices with you and hope they enrich your life as much as they have mine.

During my time in Japan, I had the privilege of living in a small town called Nara, a place rich with history and culture. Nara was the ancient capital of Japan in the 8th century, and it is surrounded by centuries-old temples, serene forests, and peaceful gardens. This environment played a huge role in shaping my understanding of wellness. I had the opportunity to observe how Japanese people approach their daily lives with mindfulness, discipline, and a deep respect for their bodies and minds.

This book is a reflection of those years spent immersed in a culture that truly knows the art of living well. The Japanese have an incredible way of blending physical, mental, and spiritual wellness into their everyday routines, and it is this harmony that I've come to appreciate and want to share with you.

In this book, I'll highlight several simple yet powerful Japanese wellness practices that you can easily incorporate into your daily routine. These principles will not only nourish your body but also help calm your mind, bringing balance and serenity to your life. Whether you're looking to improve your diet, find a deeper sense of peace, or alleviate common health concerns associated with aging, these Japanese wellness techniques are designed to help you on your journey toward better health.

I hope this guide serves as both an inspiration and a tool, helping you embrace a lifestyle of wellness and longevity, just as I have learned to do from the Japanese people I have spent time with over the years.

Let's embark on this wellness journey together, where we'll explore how small changes can lead to powerful, lasting improvements in your overall well-being.

Note: Barbara's Biography can be found at the end of the book.

Why I wrote this book for you…

In my conversations with countless individuals, I often encounter sentiments such as, "I lack time for myself," "I'm overwhelmed with busyness," "Work dominates my life, leaving no room for balance," "Something essential is absent from my life, yet its identity eludes me," "I yearn for more from life but can't manifest it," and "I feel perpetually stuck, unable to catch a break." If these resonate with you, this book may offer the crucial insights, motivation, and redirection you seek. It provides moments of tranquility, allowing your mind to quiet and listen to your intuition. These rituals have profoundly impacted my life by establishing a routine that nurtures my physical, emotional, and spiritual well-being, enabling my life goals to seamlessly fall into place and become reality. I sincerely wish the same transformation for you, which is why I present this book.

How to use this book

Embarking on a journey of self-discovery doesn't require a passport to Japan, a love for sushi, or fluency in the language. Instead, it's about immersing yourself in a time-honoured way of life that can significantly enhance your well-being on multiple levels. This book invites you to explore the rich tapestry of an ancient culture, offering practical insights that you can weave into your daily routine to enrich your life, regardless of your current circumstances.

Each chapter beckons you to embrace the fascinating aspects of this culture, encouraging you to integrate these elements into your life. Consider starting with small steps, like replacing one of your daily cups of tea with soothing green tea, experimenting with a Japanese recipe each week, dedicating a few minutes daily to meditation, setting goals that resonate with your deepest aspirations, or simply pausing to breathe between meetings.

I genuinely believe that even adopting a single ritual from this book can spark a transformation, setting off a chain reaction of positivity that propels you toward the life you've always envisioned. This book is more than a guide; it's an invitation to uncover the potential within you and cultivate a life filled with purpose and joy.

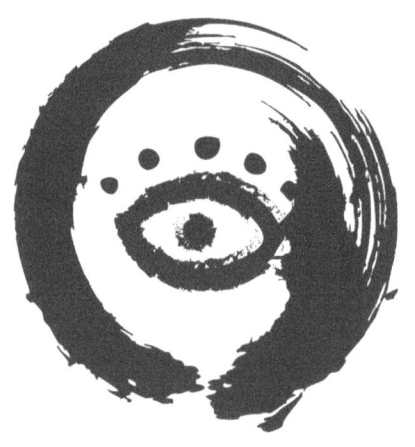

Wabi-Sabi
Admire Imperfection

CHAPTER 1

Wabi-Sabi – Admire Imperfection

Living in Nara, Japan, deeply immersed me in the philosophy of **wabi-sabi** 侘寂, a quietly powerful way of seeing the world that celebrates imperfection, impermanence, and simplicity. Though I arrived with a Western mindset that often-sought control, perfection, and constant forward momentum, Japan gradually softened those edges, teaching me to slow down, look deeper, and embrace the beauty in things as they are. I revisit this ritual when life gets a bit overwhelming and busy, and I find it soothing that I can click back into the feelings when I reflect on this principle, and I hope you will learn to too.

At first, wabi-sabi revealed itself in the most subtle ways. It was in the way tea was served in a cracked ceramic cup whose gold-filled fracture told a story. It was in the quiet pauses of conversation, the fleeting cherry blossoms, the weathered wood of a countryside shrine. These were not flaws to be fixed or moments to rush through, they were to be honoured.

In my own home, I began to shift. I embraced **kanso**, the principle of simplicity and decluttering which we will discuss in a following chapter, and I learned to appreciate the gentle wear of objects that had been loved over time. I found joy in minimalism, not as a trend, but as a form of mental and emotional spaciousness. Each season in Japan offered its own rituals, flavours, and textures as reminders to live fully in the present and allow the cycles of life to unfold naturally.

Wabi-sabi also helped me understand that healing, whether emotional, physical, or spiritual is not about returning to a previous state of "wholeness." It's about moving forward, often carrying the marks of our experiences with pride. This idea would echo later through practices like **kintsugi**, where broken pottery is repaired with gold, making it more beautiful for having been broken, another chapter for you to explore this ritual.

Living in Japan didn't just teach me about wabi-sabi, it shaped the way I live and guide others in their wellness journeys. It's the foundation for my belief that true well-being isn't found in perfection, but in presence, acceptance, and grace.

There is a quiet beauty in things that are slightly worn, a peacefulness in asymmetry, and a calm elegance in the aged. This is the spirit of *Wabi-Sabi*, a Japanese philosophy that teaches us to embrace imperfection, impermanence, and incompleteness.

Wabi-Sabi is not about fixing or improving. It's about seeing the value in what is already here, even if it's a little chipped, faded, or uneven. It asks us to move away from the modern obsession with flawless perfection and instead invites us to soften our eyes, open our hearts, and appreciate life as it is: beautifully imperfect.

Reset Your Way of Thinking

We live in a world conditioned by filters, retouching, competition, and comparison. But *Wabi-Sabi* teaches us that peace and fulfilment come when we *reset our thinking*. It's not about changing what's broken, it's about changing how we see it.

Let this be your gentle invitation to pause and reconsider your inner narrative. What if the flaws you hide are actually your unique fingerprints of experience? What if the cracks are simply proof you've lived, loved, and grown?

Trade Judgment for Acceptance

Instead of criticizing what you see, whether it's a line on your face, a scar on your skin, or a moment you wish you handled better, practice replacing judgment with acceptance.

Acceptance isn't about resignation. It's about allowing. It says, "This is how it is right now. And it's okay."

When we stop resisting, we start healing.

Forgive

One of the most powerful expressions of Wabi-Sabi is the act of forgiveness. Not just for others, but for *yourself.* Let go of the heavy stories you've been carrying, the things you think make you less-than.

Forgiveness is a profound and often underestimated wellness practice that extends far beyond emotional healing—it also supports beauty, physical health, and even longevity. Here's how forgiveness contributes to each of these areas:

Wellness

1. Reduces Stress & Anxiety:

Holding onto anger, resentment, or unresolved emotional pain triggers the body's stress response. Chronic stress elevates cortisol, a hormone that can lead to inflammation, fatigue, digestive issues, and sleep disruption. Forgiveness releases that tension, creating emotional peace and physiological balance.

2. Improves Mental Health:

Forgiveness is strongly associated with reduced symptoms of depression, anxiety, and PTSD. When you let go of resentment, you create space for clarity, compassion, and resilience.

3. Enhances Relationships:

Forgiving others (or yourself) improves communication, deepens connection, and builds trust. Strong social bonds are a well-documented pillar of long-term wellness, particularly in cultures like Japan's where community ties support emotional health.

Beauty

1. **Lowers Inflammation (Skin Health):**
Stress from unforgiveness increases systemic inflammation, which can manifest in acne, eczema, dull skin, and premature aging. By reducing this inner turmoil, forgiveness helps your skin appear clearer, brighter, and more radiant.

2. **Promotes Better Sleep (Beauty Sleep Is Real):**
People who practice forgiveness report better sleep quality. Sleep is crucial for cellular regeneration, collagen production, and that natural morning glow.

3. **Boosts Confidence & Softens Expression:**
Letting go of grudges can literally soften your face—muscle tension eases, your smile returns more freely, and your overall presence becomes more open and magnetic.

Longevity

1. **Lowers Risk of Chronic Diseases:**
Unforgiveness contributes to long-term stress, which is a risk factor for heart disease, high blood pressure, and metabolic disorders. Forgiveness, on the other hand, has been linked to improved cardiovascular health and immune function.

2. **Encourages Healthy Habits:**
When we forgive, we are more likely to care for ourselves and make nourishing choices like moving our bodies, eating well, and practicing mindfulness, because we no longer feel weighed down by emotional baggage.

3. **Supports Brain Health:**

Forgiveness has been associated with improved cognitive function in later life. Emotional well-being supports a more agile mind, better memory, and reduced risk of neurodegenerative disease.

Forgiveness is not just an act of compassion; it's an act of **liberation**. It frees your body from the chemistry of stress, your face from the tension of resentment, and your spirit from the weight of the past. In doing so, it helps you glow from within, build deeper relationships, and live a longer, more peaceful life.

You are not broken. You are becoming.

Each stumble, every heartbreak, all the missteps, they have shaped you into someone wiser, softer, and deeper. That is something to honour, not erase.

Stop Comparing

Comparison steals your joy and blinds you to your own path.

The flower does not compare itself to the tree. The moon does not envy the sun. And you have your own rhythm, timing, and brilliance.

When you let go of comparison, you allow yourself to fully live your own beautiful, imperfect story.

Simplify

Wabi-Sabi also shows up in simplicity.

In a world of more, it gently reminds us that less often brings more clarity. More peace. More room to breathe, instead of more stuff gathering dust in your home.

Declutter your home. Declutter your schedule. Declutter your expectations, yes, that's a good one, right!

Decluttering expectations is just as important as decluttering your home or workspace, it frees up mental and emotional space so you can live with more peace, authenticity, and presence. Here's how to do it mindfully and effectively:

How to Declutter Expectations

1. **Become Aware of Hidden Expectations**

Many expectations operate under the surface:

- "I should have achieved more by now."
- "They should understand how I feel."
- "Life should look a certain way."

Practice:

Take a quiet moment and journal your current frustrations. Then ask, *"What expectation is behind this?"* You'll start to uncover internal "rules" you didn't even realize were shaping your mood and choices.

2. Identify Which Expectations Are Serving You

Not all expectations are bad. Some can motivate or create structure—but others only create pressure or disappointment.

Try This:

For each major expectation, ask:

- Is this realistic?
- Is this mine, or someone else's (family, culture, social media)?
- Does this help me grow, or keep me stuck?

Let go of the ones that feel heavy, outdated, or externally imposed.

3. Replace "Should" with "Could"

Language reveals a lot about our inner state. "Should" often implies guilt or unmet pressure. "Could" invites possibility and flexibility.

Shift the mindset:

- "I should be more productive" → "I *could* choose one thing that matters today."
- "They should text me back" → "They *could* be going through something I don't know about."

4. **Let Go of Timeline Pressure**

We often expect life to unfold in a certain order—by a certain age or deadline. This can lead to unnecessary comparison and stress.

Reframe:

Life is not a checklist. It's a flow. Trust your own timing, even if it doesn't look like anyone else's.

5. **Practice Wabi-Sabi Thinking**

From Japanese philosophy, *wabi-sabi* is the acceptance of imperfection, impermanence, and incompleteness. Life is sometimes messy and it's often evolving and that's beautiful.

Ask:

Can I find grace and beauty in how things are, rather than how I expected them to be?

6. **Create Space for the Unexpected**

When we drop rigid expectations, we open ourselves to surprise, spontaneity, and joy. Life becomes less about controlling outcomes and more about embracing what is.

Practice:

Leave part of your day unscheduled. Try saying "yes" to something spontaneous. Let go of needing to know how things will turn out.

Decluttering expectations is a practice of freedom. It invites you to meet life where it is, not where you think it *should* be. When you drop the pressure of control, you gain the peace of presence.

Find the sacred in the simple. A quiet cup of tea. A handwritten note. A walk without headphones.

Simplicity brings space. And space brings truth.

Work on Self-Acceptance

Self-acceptance isn't a destination; it's a practice.

It's whispering, "I'm enough" even when the world is shouting "more." It's showing up for yourself with compassion. It's giving yourself grace when you fall short.

Celebrate your quirks. Honour your emotions. Embrace your pace.

Because the more you accept yourself, the more space you create for growth.

Look at Wisdom as Beauty

We've been taught to revere youth, but Wabi-Sabi teaches us to revere *experience*.

A wrinkle can be a laugh line. A scar can be a survival story. A grey hair can be a crown of wisdom.

Beauty is not just what we see, it's what we *know*, what we've *lived*, and how we *love*.

Final Thought

Wabi-Sabi is not a trend. It's a mindset. A gentle shift from striving to being, from fixing to seeing, from perfection to presence.

When you learn to admire imperfection in yourself, in others, and in life, you open the door to peace, authenticity, and joy.

Let the cracks show. Let the real in.

Because sometimes, the most beautiful things are the ones that are just a little bit worn.

Now you have a choice to continue reading, or turn to the Journal prompt session that acts as a little workbook for your thoughts and actions, so you can implement the learnings, realisations and acknowledgements of where we can make small improvements in our life that reflect the rituals of longevity.

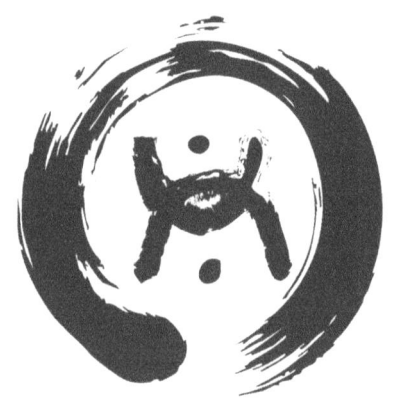

Gaman
Live with Great Resilience

CHAPTER 2

Gaman – Live with Great Resilience

In the Japanese tradition, *Gaman* (我慢) is a quiet strength, a cultural cornerstone that reflects the power of endurance, patience and self-control, especially during life's storms. It is not about pretending everything is okay. It's about staying grounded even when the winds of life threaten to knock you down.

To *live with great resilience* doesn't mean never breaking, it means bending without falling. It means carrying yourself with dignity through discomfort, adapting when needed, and rising again and again.

Take Action

Resilience is not passive. *Gaman* asks you to take action, deliberate, take mindful steps forward, no matter how small.

Do one thing today that strengthens your tomorrow.

Start with a walk. Clean one drawer. Make one healthy meal. Resilience is built in the doing, not in the waiting.

Eat Fresh

The body fuels the mind. Eating clean, fresh, whole foods nourishes more than your physical health, it stabilizes your emotions, your focus, your energy.

Choose seasonal vegetables. Add colour to your plate. Avoid processed quick fixes. This is resilience in action: making nourishing choices when it's easier to settle for less.

Eat to honour your strength and read more about the principles of a Japanese diet in chapter 3 and be inspired to try some new food ingredients in your meals that are commonly used to nourish the body the Japanese way.

Cut Back

Simplify. Resilience grows when there's space to breathe.

Cut back on things that drain you like sugar, screen time, late nights, negative conversations. Gaman is not about restriction; it's about *refinement*. Keep what builds you. Release what breaks you.

Decluttering your environment often begins by decluttering your choices.

Get Moving

Movement is medicine. Whether it's a brisk walk, dancing in your kitchen, or stretching with intention, moving your body moves your spirit.

You don't need to run a marathon. Just move with purpose. Let motion create momentum. A resilient body supports a resilient mind.

Socialize in Real Life

True resilience is not built in isolation. *Gaman* doesn't mean you must endure everything alone.

Spend time with people who lift you. Meet a friend for tea. Call someone you love. Share a laugh. Be present with others.

Real connection builds emotional immunity. It reminds you that you're never alone in your struggles.

Work Out

Exercise isn't just about physique; it's about mindset as well.

It teaches you discipline, persistence, and the ability to push through when it's uncomfortable. These are the same muscles you'll flex when life gets hard.

Commit to a routine that works for *you*. Show up, sweat it out, and let your body mirror your mental strength.

Meditate

When the world gets loud, go inward.

Meditation is not about silencing thoughts; it's about not letting them control you. It builds inner stillness, clarity, and the space to respond instead of reacting.

Even five minutes a day of breathwork or mindful silence can rewire your resilience.

Make Peace

Let go of grudges. Forgive what no longer serves you. Gaman teaches emotional fortitude through peace, not through resistance. Re-read about forgiveness in chapter one if this is an area that instinctively you feel needs attention.

Peace is power. It frees up energy you can use to heal, create, and move forward.

Letting go doesn't mean forgetting. It means choosing your freedom.

Stay the Course

Resilience is a practice, not a personality trait.

You won't always feel strong. That's okay. What matters is that you stay the course, and you rest when needed, cry when needed, pause when needed, but *don't quit on yourself*, ever!

Life's trials will test you. Gaman says: *You are greater than your challenge.*

Final Thought

Resilience is quiet. It's not flashy or loud. It doesn't seek praise. It shows up every day in small ways, in your food, your thoughts, your choices, and your actions.

Gaman is not just surviving. It's enduring with grace. It's enduring with integrity. It's enduring with hope.

Live with great resilience. Not because it's easy, but because you can.

If you feel compelled to journal, then head over to the journal prompts for this chapter and pour your thoughts, feelings and actions onto paper. Then once poured out, you can acknowledge them, come to terms with them, and put actions in place to deal with them.

三

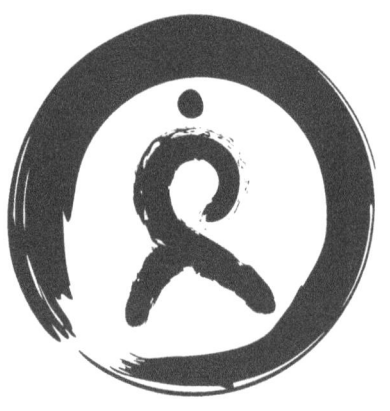

Eiyoshoku
Nourish Your Body

CHAPTER 3

Eiyoshoku – Nourish Your Body

Inspired by Japan: The Birth of Nutrichef

Living in Japan was a transformative chapter in my life. Surrounded by a culture that reveres balance, mindfulness, and nature, not just in art and design, but also in food and I found myself inspired every single day. The way meals were prepared with care, the use of fresh, seasonal ingredients, the smaller portions, and the emphasis on gut-friendly foods like fermented miso paste, vegetables and grains, it all started to make perfect sense. More importantly, I *felt* amazing. My energy increased, my cravings disappeared, my weight normalised, my skin improved, and I experienced a deep sense of wellness that I'd never truly felt before.

This wasn't just about what was on the plate, it was about a way of life. Food was medicine. Food was a ritual. Food was respect for the body and for my future self, in prevention of food related illnesses like heart disease, diabetes and even some cancers are food related.

When I returned to the UK after living ten years in in Nara, on a triangle between Oaka and Kyoto, I knew I couldn't leave that wisdom behind. In 2004, I founded **Nutrichef**, a healthy meal delivery company rooted in those Japanese principles: quality ingredients, mindful preparation, and nourishing the body from the inside out. My mission was simple but profound; to help people experience the same vitality and wellbeing I had discovered through food.

Over the 12 years I helmed Nutrichef, I had the privilege of fuelling thousands of customers across the UK like Olympic and professional athletes, busy professionals, new parents, and anyone eager to feel better, think clearer, lose weight and live longer through the power of food. Every menu was carefully curated, not just for taste but for purpose. We helped people lose weight, manage inflammation, improve digestion, and simply feel *more alive*.

Nutrichef wasn't just a business, it was a movement, from healthy meals delivered to healthy snacks sold in supermarkets and online. Its roots were planted in the heart of Japanese wellness traditions that continue to shape my life and philosophy today.

I founded and led Nutrichef from 2004 to 2015, when it was sold in a 2 year buy out, but I personally have continued the principles at home raising my family and entertaining friends with amazing Japanese food principles and delicious recipes.

In Japanese culture, Eiyoshoku (栄養食) means "nutritional food" but more than just eating for sustenance, it embodies the philosophy of food as medicine, prevention over cure, and respect for what nourishes us. The Japanese diet is one of the most celebrated globally for its health benefits, known for supporting longevity, vitality, and graceful aging.

This chapter invites you to not only look at *what* you eat but *how* you eat to nourish your body with intention, balance, and gratitude.

The Principles of a Japanese Diet

1. Seasonal and Local Ingredients

Nature knows best. Traditional Japanese meals highlight seasonal produce, eaten at the peak of freshness. From spring bamboo shoots to autumn chestnuts, this approach is rooted in the concept of *shun*, which is eating foods when they are most vibrant and nutritious. I have fond memories of grocery shopping for seasonal sweet potatoes, medicinal mushrooms like reishii and maitake mushrooms, seasonal gingko nuts and fresh peas in the pods. My mouth is starting to water just thinking about it.

Ask yourself: *Am I eating what nature is offering right now?*

2. Balanced Variety in Small Portions

A typical Japanese meal includes multiple small dishes, rather than one large plate. This offers a variety of different colours, textures, and nutrients all without overeating. Meals might consist of a bowl of rice, miso soup, pickled vegetables, grilled fish, and some steamed greens.

It's not about restriction, but harmony and balance.

3. Mostly Plant-Based, With Fish

The traditional Japanese diet is rich in vegetables, seaweed, tofu, rice, and legumes, with moderate amounts of fish and minimal red meat or dairy. Fermented foods like miso, natto, and pickles help support gut health, digestion, and immunity.

4. Eat Until 80% Full – *'Hara Hachi Bu'*

This powerful principle from Okinawan culture teaches us to stop eating before we are completely full. The idea is to avoid overeating and give the body time to digest slowly. This habit is linked to longevity and maintaining a healthy weight.

Mindful eating is central to Japanese wellness.

5. Soup with Every Meal

A bowl of warm, mineral-rich miso soup is common at breakfast, lunch, and dinner. Light broths hydrate, aid digestion, and offer umami satisfaction without heaviness. It's comfort in a cup. Umami is actually considered the fifth basic taste, alongside sweet, sour, salty, and bitter.

6. Green Tea as a Ritual

Green tea is more than a beverage in Japan; it's a moment of pause. Rich in antioxidants, it supports metabolism and calm alertness. Replacing sugary drinks with green tea is a small, nourishing act of self-care. I personally start my morning with a cup of green tea; that's part of my morning ritual.

7. Minimal Processing, Maximum Respect

Meals are minimally processed, cooked gently (steamed, simmered, grilled), and seasoned lightly to let the natural flavours shine. There's a deep respect for ingredients, for what the earth, sea, and sky provide.

8. Presentation Matters

The Japanese believe that *we eat with our eyes first.* Meals are arranged artfully and thoughtfully. Beauty on the plate reflects gratitude and mindfulness, which enhances digestion and satisfaction. I must confess, I have fallen in love with Japanese dishes, pottery, lacquerware and chopsticks. I adore arranging Japanese delicacies in beautifully crafted pottery dishes in all shapes, sizes and designs.

Your Eiyoshoku Practice Starts Here

To nourish your body the Eiyoshoku way:

- Choose whole, seasonal foods.
- Add more fermented and plant-based ingredients.
- Practice *'hara hachi bu'* — slow down, eat mindfully, and honour fullness and stop eating when you feel 80% full.
- Sip warm broth (seaweed broth, miso broth, bone broth or tea instead of cold drinks.
- Treat meals as a ritual, not a rush.

Shojin Ryori — The Cuisine of Devotion

Shojin ryori (精進料理), meaning "food of devotion," is the traditional vegetarian cuisine practiced for centuries by Buddhist monks in Japan. Rooted in the principles of compassion, mindfulness, and respect for all living beings, this style of cooking reflects a deep spiritual connection between food and life.

At its heart, *shojin ryori* is about simplicity and harmony. It celebrates the natural flavours of seasonal, plant-based ingredients and nothing is wasted as every part of a vegetable, from root to leaf, is thoughtfully used. Preparing and eating *shojin ryori* is more than nourishment; it is a meditative act of gratitude, presence, and reverence.

You don't need to be a monk to enjoy the benefits of *shojin ryori*. Its minimal yet elegant recipes and intentional approach make it a beautiful practice to bring into your own home kitchen. It's a perfect companion to the Japanese dietary principles discussed earlier in this book, offering a deeper way to slow down, eat clean, and live well.

Omakase — The Art of Trust in Dining

Not in the mood to cook? There's a beautiful Japanese dining tradition that turns even eating out into an experience of connection and mindfulness.

Omakase (お任せ), meaning "I'll leave it up to you," is a style of dining where the chef selects and serves a curated sequence of dishes based on the freshest available ingredients. Often experienced at sushi bars, *omakase* is a culinary journey that's built on trust and mutual respect, and you place yourself entirely in the hands of the chef, allowing their expertise and intuition to guide your meal.

If you choose to enjoy an *omakase* experience, try to find a restaurant that honours the principles of balance and clean eating with fresh, seasonal ingredients, minimal processing, and thoughtful presentation. When done mindfully, *omakase* dining becomes a celebration of nature, skill, and sensory appreciation. I have done this many times, and always come away from this experience inspired,

The Okinawa Diet

The Okinawa Diet is one of the most well-known and studied dietary patterns from the Blue Zones, areas of the world where people live the longest, healthiest lives. Okinawa, a Japanese island located in the southern part of the country, has gained international attention for its high number of centenarians (people aged 100 or older) and for the overall longevity and health of its population.

The Okinawa diet is deeply linked to the island's culture and the healthy lifestyle of its residents. It emphasizes a balance of whole foods, a variety of plant-based ingredients, and certain eating practices that contribute to longevity and disease prevention.

Okinawa and the Science of Longevity

Research into the diets of the Okinawan people has provided a wealth of scientific insights into how certain dietary patterns can contribute to longevity and a reduction in age-related diseases. Here are some of the key scientific findings:

1. Oxidative Stress and Antioxidants:
   - The Okinawan diet is rich in antioxidants that help combat oxidative stress, a process where free radicals damage cells, contributing to aging and diseases like cancer and cardiovascular conditions. The abundance of vegetables, fruits, and plant-based foods in the Okinawan diet provides ample antioxidants that protect the body from these harmful effects.
   - Purple sweet potatoes and green tea, two staples in the Okinawan diet, are especially high in antioxidants like anthocyanins and catechins, which reduce inflammation and cellular damage.
2. Caloric Restriction and Longevity:
   - Studies have shown that caloric restriction (reducing the intake of calories without malnutrition) is one of the most effective ways to extend lifespan in animals and humans. Okinawans naturally practice caloric restriction due to their culture of portion control and mindful eating practices like Hara Hachi Bu. This has been linked to improved metabolic function, reduced oxidative stress, and a lower risk of diseases like cancer and heart disease.

- o The Okinawan population has one of the lowest incidences of age-related diseases and the highest proportion of centenarians in the world. Studies on caloric restriction in animals show that it can delay the aging process and extend lifespan, possibly by slowing down cellular damage and inflammation.
3. Healthy Gut Microbiome:
   - o A diverse diet rich in fibre from vegetables, legumes, and fermented foods (such as miso and pickled vegetables) promotes a healthy gut microbiome. A healthy gut microbiome is associated with improved immune function, reduced inflammation, and lower risks of metabolic diseases, which contribute to longevity.
   - o The gut-brain axis, the connection between the gut and the brain has also been linked to mental health and cognitive function, areas where Okinawans appear to excel. Okinawans tend to have lower rates of cognitive decline and Alzheimer's disease, possibly due to their diet, active lifestyle, and strong social connections.
4. Heart Health and Omega-3 Fatty Acids:
   - o Okinawans consume a diet high in omega-3 fatty acids, which are beneficial for heart health. Studies have shown that omega-3s help reduce inflammation, lower blood pressure, and reduce the risk of heart disease.
   - o Additionally, Okinawan diets are low in processed foods and high in plant-based foods, which also help maintain healthy cholesterol levels and reduce the risk of heart disease.

5. Low Incidence of Chronic Diseases:
   o The combination of a nutrient-dense, low-calorie diet and physical activity in Okinawa has led to lower rates of chronic diseases such as type 2 diabetes, obesity, and hypertension. The Okinawan diet's emphasis on eating whole, unprocessed foods is thought to be a significant factor in this reduced disease risk.

The Okinawa diet is a powerful example of how dietary habits, combined with a culture of mindfulness, respect for nature, and social support, can promote longevity and health. By focusing on whole, nutrient-dense foods, practicing portion control, and embracing traditional eating habits, the Okinawan population has become a model of health and vitality in old age. Scientific research continues to confirm that many of the principles followed by Okinawans, such as caloric restriction, antioxidant-rich foods, and omega-3 fatty acids, contribute significantly to their long, healthy lives.

Adopting elements of the Okinawa diet can be a step toward improving your own health and longevity and can lead to a more balanced and nourishing lifestyle.

If you're feeling hungry, then now is the time to journey and start meal planning with some additions of healthy Japanese foods and recipes. Head over to chapter 26 journal prompts and also get some inspiration with some easy to cook Japanese recipes in chapter 27.

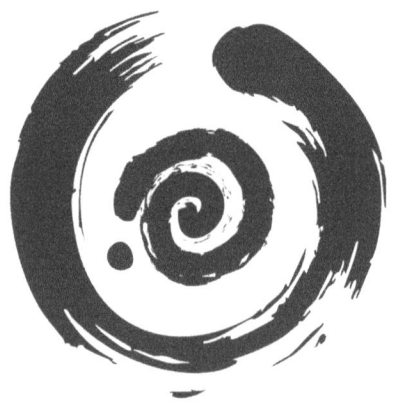

Kiotsukete
Learn to Take Care

CHAPTER 4

Kiotsukete – Learn to Take Care

In Japanese, *Kiotsukete* (気をつけて) is often said when parting ways as it means "take care." But this simple phrase holds a deeper philosophy: a reminder to be mindful, protective, and nurturing of both self and others. In today's fast-paced world, true care often takes a backseat to productivity and distraction and now is the time to reclaim it.

1. Trust Yourself

Care begins with trust, especially self-trust. We spend so much time seeking advice, affirmation, and permission from others that we can forget we hold wisdom within. Trust that quiet voice inside. Trust your ability to choose what's right for your mind, body, and soul. Trust that you're doing your best and that your best is enough.

"Your inner voice is the compass you were born with. Listen."

2. Listen to Your Intuition

Our intuition is our built-in guide. It often whispers rather than shouts, so we must create quiet moments to hear it. This could mean journaling, meditating, walking without a podcast or music on your earphones, or simply sitting with a decision. When we truly listen, our intuition leads us toward the people, places, and choices that support our wellbeing.

3. Be at One with Nature

Nature heals, balances, and grounds us. It teaches rhythm, impermanence, and beauty. Make time to step outside, even briefly. Notice the breeze, the shifting clouds, or the way the earth smells after rain. Let nature's calm enter your body. Taking care of yourself is easier when you're reminded of your place in a larger, living system.

4. Eat for Care

Eating is one of the most intimate ways we care for ourselves. Ask yourself not just *what* you're eating, but *why*. Choose foods that nourish, energize, and respect your body's needs. Enjoy meals without rush. Hydrate. Slow down. Make eating a ritual of self-love. Re-read chapter 3, Eiyoshoku if more inspiration is needed to nourish your body.

5. Move with Intention

Movement is a gift, not a punishment. Walk, stretch, dance, swim, breathe. Move not to shrink yourself, but to feel more alive within your body. Movement should feel like kindness, not a chore. I often see people in the gym pushing themselves, strained faces, all to lose weight. Moving with intention and having a multi-faceted weight loss regime will support your weight transformation with faster and longer-lasting benefits and results.

6. Say No with Love

Caring for yourself means setting boundaries. Not everything deserves your "yes." Say no so that your yeses are more powerful and meaningful. Saying no doesn't mean rejecting others, it means choosing what protects your energy, your times, your value.

Setting and maintaining boundaries is essential for personal wellbeing and healthy relationships. Here are a few easy tips to help you establish and uphold boundaries effectively:

1. Know Your Limits: Take time to reflect on your values, needs, and limits. Understanding what is acceptable and what is not will help you communicate your boundaries clearly.
2. Communicate Clearly: Use straightforward and assertive language when expressing your boundaries. Be specific about what you need and why it's important to you.
3. Be Consistent: Consistency is key to maintaining boundaries. Stick to your limits and reinforce them, when necessary, even if it's challenging.

4. Practice Saying No: It's okay to say no without feeling guilty. Practice assertive ways to decline requests that don't align with your boundaries or priorities.

5. Use "I" Statements: When discussing boundaries, use "I" statements to express your feelings and needs. For example, "I feel overwhelmed when..." or "I need time to recharge."

6. Start Small: If setting boundaries feels daunting, start with small, manageable ones. Gradually work your way up to more significant boundaries as you gain confidence.

7. Be Mindful of Your Energy: Pay attention to how interactions and commitments affect your energy levels. Set boundaries that protect your time and energy.

8. Seek Support: If you're struggling to set or maintain boundaries, seek support from friends, family, or a therapist. They can offer guidance and encouragement.

9. Respect Others' Boundaries: Just as you set your own boundaries, respect the boundaries of others. This mutual respect fosters healthier relationships.

10. Reflect and Adjust: Regularly reflect on your boundaries and adjust them as needed. Life changes, and your boundaries may need to evolve accordingly.

By implementing these tips, you can create a balanced and fulfilling life that honours your needs and promotes positive relationships.

7. Say Yes to Joy

Self-care isn't only about detox teas and bubble baths, it's also about laughter, music, silliness, adventure, and rest. Let joy be part of your care practice. It nourishes just as deeply as discipline.

8. Get the Sleep You Need

Rest is not a luxury. It's foundational. Prioritize quality sleep by creating an evening routine, limiting screen time, and winding down with intention. Let your body recover, so your mind can reset. Look at your bedroom environment from bedding, to lighting, to temperature to electromagnetic waves. A deeper dive into sleep regime is for you to research if this area needs support, but here's a few tips to get started with:

Establishing a good nighttime routine can significantly improve the quality of your sleep. Here are a few tips to help you create a better sleep routine:

1. **Consistent Sleep Schedule:** Try to go to bed and wake up at the same time every day, even on weekends. Consistency reinforces your body's natural sleep-wake cycle.
2. **Create a Relaxing Bedtime Routine:** Engage in calming activities before bed, such as reading, taking a warm bath, or practicing meditation. This helps signal to your body that it's time to wind down.
3. **Limit Screen Time:** Reduce exposure to screens (phones, tablets, computers, TVs) at least an hour

before bed. The blue light emitted by screens can interfere with your ability to fall asleep.

4. **Comfortable Sleep Environment:** Ensure your bedroom is conducive to sleep. Keep the room cool, dark, and quiet. Consider using blackout curtains, earplugs, or a white noise machine if needed.

5. **Mind Your Diet:** Avoid large meals, caffeine, and alcohol close to bedtime. These can disrupt your sleep or make it harder to fall asleep.

6. **Physical Activity:** Regular physical activity can help you fall asleep faster and enjoy deeper sleep. However, try to avoid vigorous exercise close to bedtime.

7. **Manage Stress:** Practice relaxation techniques such as deep breathing, progressive muscle relaxation, or journaling to manage stress and anxiety before bed.

8. **Limit Naps:** If you nap during the day, keep it short (20-30 minutes) and avoid napping late in the afternoon to prevent interference with nighttime sleep.

9. **Comfortable Bedding:** Invest in a comfortable mattress and pillows that support restful sleep. Your bedding should be inviting and conducive to relaxation.

10. **Avoid Clock-Watching:** If you find yourself unable to sleep, avoid watching the clock. This can increase anxiety and make it harder to fall asleep.

By incorporating these tips into your nightly routine, you can create an environment and habits that promote restful and rejuvenating sleep.

9. Nurture Your Relationships

Take care of the people who take care of you. A simple message, shared tea, or act of presence can strengthen bonds. Relationships are part of our wellbeing ecosystem. Water them, water them daily!

10. Do It Daily

Care is not something you do once in a while. It's a lifestyle. Tiny daily decisions shape your wellbeing far more than one-off gestures. Start each day by asking, *"How can I care for myself today?"*

Kiotsukete: A Way of Life

Taking care of yourself is not selfish. It's foundational. When we care for ourselves, mindfully and consistently, we become more able to care for others, face challenges, and enjoy life fully. Start where you are, with what you have, and give yourself the same tenderness you'd give to someone you deeply love.

If you have a few minutes, turn over to the journal prompts for Kiostukete.

Taking action is a fundamental step in creating results because it transforms ideas and intentions into tangible outcomes. Here's why taking action is so effective:

1. **Bridges the Gap:** Action bridges the gap between where you are and where you want to be. It moves you from planning and dreaming to doing and achieving.

2. **Builds Momentum:** Once you start taking action, even small steps can build momentum. This momentum makes it easier to continue moving forward and tackling larger tasks.

3. **Creates Opportunities:** By taking action, you open yourself up to new opportunities and experiences that you might not have encountered otherwise. Action often leads to unexpected paths and possibilities.

4. **Facilitates Learning:** Action provides real-world feedback and learning experiences. You gain insights and knowledge that can only come from doing, allowing you to adjust and improve your approach.

5. **Overcomes Fear and Procrastination:** Taking action helps overcome fear and procrastination by shifting focus from potential obstacles to tangible progress. It builds confidence and reduces anxiety.

6. **Transforms Ideas into Reality:** Ideas remain abstract until action is taken. By acting on your ideas, you bring them into the real world, making them concrete and achievable.

7. **Demonstrates Commitment:** Taking action shows commitment to your goals and values. It signals to yourself and others that you are serious about achieving your objectives.

8. **Generates Results:** Ultimately, action is what generates results. Without action, goals remain unfulfilled, and potential remains untapped.

By taking action, you set the stage for growth, achievement, and success. It's the catalyst that turns aspirations into accomplishments and dreams into reality. Ganbatte …. The next chapter explains Ganbatte!

Remember if you're inspired by journaling, no wis your chance, so turn to chapter 26 for journal prompts to take this topic deeper.

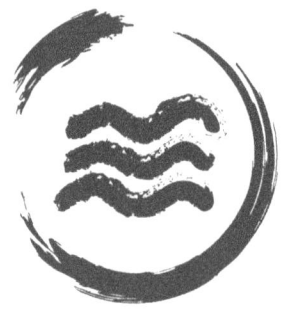

Ganbatte
Always Do Your Best by Hanging In There

CHAPTER 5

Ganbatte – Always Do Your Best by Hanging in There

"Ganbatte" がんばって is a powerful Japanese expression that goes beyond simply doing your best, it's about perseverance, grit, and giving your full effort no matter the challenge. It means to show up, dig deep, and push through even when it's hard. It's not perfection, it's persistence. It's about staying the course with heart and dignity.

In Japanese culture, the phrase *"Ganbatte!"* is a rallying cry. It means *"do your best,"* but it carries a weight much deeper than effort alone. It's a reminder to endure with dignity, to press forward with all your heart, and to rise with grace when life pushes you down, and we're all supporting along the way!

This chapter is a celebration of inner strength, the kind that shows up in early mornings, tough conversations, honest mistakes, and unwavering dedication. *Ganbatte* is about staying the course, not because it's easy, but because it matters.

Embrace the Struggle

Struggle is not failure. It is the sculptor of strength. Every time you choose to keep going, despite discomfort, you train resilience. There is beauty in not giving up, no matter how slowly you move, you're still moving forward.

"The bamboo that bends is stronger than the oak that resists." – Japanese Proverb

Let go of perfection. Let go of the need for constant ease. Embrace the messy, the challenging, and the uncomfortable. These moments are where your best self is born.

Give It Your All

Doing your best doesn't mean being perfect. It means bringing the fullness of who you are to the task at hand. It means showing up wholeheartedly, staying present, and honouring your potential.

Ask yourself: "Did I bring my full attention? Did I act with integrity? Did I try, even when no one was watching?" That is the true measure of *Ganbatte*.

Be on Time

Punctuality is not just about clocks. It's a reflection of commitment, respect, and self-discipline. Being on time shows others, and yourself, that you value your word and the energy of others. It's a small habit that creates lasting trust.

Be Yourself

There is no substitute for authenticity. Your unique presence, talents, and voice are your greatest assets. Don't dilute them. The world needs more real people, imperfect, human, and honest. Do your best by being unapologetically yourself.

Wish Others the Best

One of the most graceful acts of strength is to wish others well, especially when you're struggling yourself. *Ganbatte* isn't a competition; it's a shared experience. Uplifting others even in your own hard times builds compassion, unity, and a sense of purpose.

Be Honest

To do your best means to live with truth. Speak it. Own it. Honour it. Honesty keeps your inner world in alignment with your outer actions. It's the glue that holds integrity together and integrity is the foundation of lasting strength.

Final Thought

Ganbatte is not about grand gestures. It's about quiet endurance, daily efforts, and fierce belief in the value of persistence. Keep showing up. Keep believing. And above all, never give up.

Here's how "ganbatte" can relate to the concept of longevity:

1. **Perseverance in Health:** The mindset of "ganbatte" encourages individuals to persist in their health and

wellness efforts, even when faced with challenges. This perseverance can lead to healthier lifestyle choices and a commitment to long-term well-being.

2. **Resilience in Adversity:** Longevity is not just about physical health but also mental and emotional resilience. "Ganbatte" inspires people to remain strong and positive in the face of life's adversities, contributing to overall longevity.

3. **Continuous Improvement:** The spirit of "ganbatte" aligns with the idea of continuous self-improvement and lifelong learning, both of which are important for maintaining cognitive health and vitality as we age.

4. **Community Support:** "Ganbatte" is often used to encourage others, fostering a sense of community and support. Strong social connections are linked to longer, healthier lives, as they provide emotional support and reduce stress.

5. **Mindful Living:** By embracing "ganbatte," individuals may approach each day with mindfulness and intention, focusing on doing their best in every aspect of life. This mindful approach can enhance the quality of life and contribute to longevity.

In essence, "ganbatte" embodies qualities that promote a fulfilling and resilient life, which are key components of longevity. By adopting this mindset, individuals can enhance their well-being and increase their chances of living a long, healthy life.

Now, head over to the journal prompt for Ganbatte, and explore the feelings, thoughts and actions that come to mind.

六

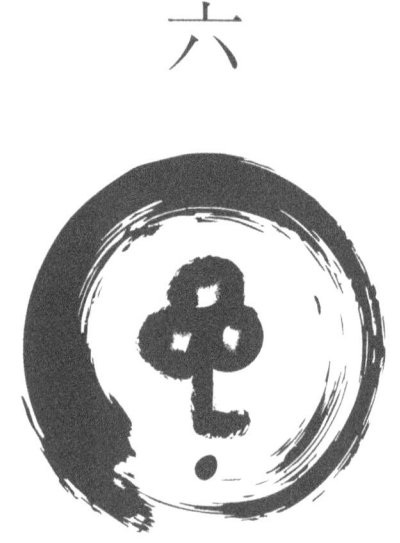

Kaizen
Continuously Improve

CHAPTER 6

Kaizen – Continuously Improve

In life, there is a constant opportunity for growth, learning, and improvement. The Japanese principle of *Kaizen* 改善 is built upon the concept of continuous, incremental improvement. Unlike big, often overwhelming changes, *Kaizen* teaches us that small steps taken consistently can lead to monumental transformations over time. It's about the mindset of never stopping the process of refining ourselves, our work, and our lives.

At its core, *Kaizen* is more than just a way to improve; it's about cultivating a lifestyle that embraces progress, no matter how small the step. Through continuous improvement, we can achieve higher levels of success, satisfaction, and fulfilment.

1. The Power of Small Steps

One of the most remarkable aspects of *Kaizen* is its emphasis on small, steady steps. Rather than setting lofty goals that may feel intimidating, *Kaizen* encourages us to focus on making slight but consistent changes every day. Over time, these changes build up, leading to substantial growth.

It's important to remember that improvement doesn't always require dramatic shifts. The beauty of *Kaizen* is that tiny steps, compounded day by day, can create great results. This is especially helpful for those looking to make lasting changes that won't overwhelm them.

2. Lifelong Learning

With *Kaizen*, we embrace the fact that growth is a lifelong pursuit. There's always room to learn, grow, and refine skills, no matter how much experience we have. This mindset encourages us to continuously seek new knowledge, experiences, and ways to improve our capabilities.

Whether it's taking a course, reading a book, seeking feedback, or experimenting with new ideas, *Kaizen* encourages us to stay curious and open to learning. By doing so, we expand our minds, increase our effectiveness, and evolve into better versions of ourselves.

3. Embracing Failure as a Stepping Stone

Kaizen teaches us to look at failure not as a setback, but as a natural part of the process. We learn from our mistakes, and each misstep offers valuable insight for our growth. In fact, the idea of "failing forward" is integral to *Kaizen*. Each time we fail, we are given the opportunity to make adjustments and come back stronger.

By embracing failure as an essential aspect of improvement, we reduce the fear of failure, freeing ourselves to experiment, grow, and try new things. It helps us maintain the persistence needed for continuous development.

4. Improving Every Aspect of Life

Kaizen isn't limited to just one part of your life. This principle can be applied to every area, from work to health, relationships, hobbies, and personal growth. Whether you're aiming to be more productive at work, healthier in your personal life, or more mindful in your relationships, *Kaizen* offers a simple, sustainable approach to improvement.

For instance, in the workplace, small improvements in processes can lead to greater productivity and efficiency. At home, simple lifestyle changes, like decluttering your space or establishing a new family routine, can improve your overall quality of life.

5. Self-Awareness and Reflection

A key component of *Kaizen* is constant self-assessment. It's important to reflect on your actions, habits, and behaviours regularly to identify where improvement is needed. This self-awareness is crucial to understanding where you are and where you want to be.

To practice self-awareness, set aside time for reflection each day or week. Ask yourself questions like: What worked well today? What could I improve tomorrow? How can I continue progressing? This reflective process ensures you are constantly learning from your experiences and adjusting your approach to be better. Journalling with prompts in this book can also support this.

6. Simplifying for Greater Impact

Another crucial aspect of *Kaizen* is the elimination of waste. By simplifying processes and focusing on what truly matters, you can create more impact with less effort. This principle applies not only to work but to all areas of life.

For example, in daily life, simplifying your routine can make your day more productive and less stressful. In work, streamlining tasks and cutting out unnecessary steps can boost efficiency. By continually refining the way you do things, you make life easier and more effective.

7. Mindset for Success

The *Kaizen* mindset is essential for long-term success. It encourages you to view challenges as opportunities and small wins as important milestones. A *Kaizen* approach fosters a positive, growth-oriented mindset that helps you stay motivated and engaged with the process of self-improvement.

Through consistent small changes, you will eventually reach your larger goals. But more importantly, *Kaizen* teaches you to enjoy the journey, recognizing that personal growth is a fulfilling experience in and of itself.

Putting Kaizen into Practice

1. Start Small:

Pick one area of your life where you want to improve and take a small, simple step to get started. Whether it's improving your health, becoming more productive, or learning a new skill, choose one thing and focus on making tiny improvements each day.

2. Reflect Daily:

End each day with a quick reflection. Ask yourself what went well and where you could improve. This reflection helps reinforce the habit of continuous improvement and keeps you on track.

3. Embrace Continuous Learning:

Make learning a regular part of your life. Whether it's through reading, taking courses, or seeking feedback, commit to learning something new each day. This constant growth keeps you adaptable and open to new opportunities.

4. Be Patient:

Change doesn't happen overnight. Trust the process of continuous improvement and be patient with yourself as you gradually make progress. With time, those small steps will lead to significant transformation.

Kaizen is more than just a practice; it's a way of living. It teaches us that continuous improvement, no matter how small, can lead to profound growth. By embracing the principles of *Kaizen*, we can create a life that is always evolving and improving, allowing us to achieve our personal and professional goals while fostering a deeper sense of fulfilment.

Remember, *Kaizen* is about progress, not perfection. And with each small step, you're becoming a better, more refined version of yourself. This approach can significantly support longevity in several ways:

1. **Sustainable Lifestyle Changes:** Kaizen encourages making small, manageable changes rather than drastic overhauls. This approach can lead to sustainable lifestyle habits that promote long-term health and well-being, such as gradually improving diet, exercise, and sleep routines.

2. **Stress Reduction:** By focusing on incremental improvements, kaizen reduces the pressure and stress associated with trying to achieve perfection quickly. Lower stress levels are associated with better health outcomes and increased longevity.

3. **Enhanced Mental Agility:** The practice of kaizen involves continuous learning and adaptation, which keeps the mind active and engaged. This mental agility can help maintain cognitive function and reduce the risk of age-related cognitive decline.

4. **Improved Problem-Solving:** Kaizen fosters a proactive approach to problem-solving, encouraging individuals to identify and address issues before

they become significant. This mindset can lead to better health management and prevention of chronic conditions.

5. **Increased Motivation and Satisfaction:** The sense of accomplishment from achieving small goals can boost motivation and satisfaction. This positive reinforcement encourages ongoing efforts to improve health and well-being, contributing to a longer, more fulfilling life.

6. **Community and Collaboration:** Kaizen often involves teamwork and collaboration, fostering strong social connections. Social engagement is a key factor in longevity, as it provides emotional support and reduces feelings of isolation.

By integrating the principles of kaizen into daily life, individuals can create a balanced and proactive approach to health and longevity, focusing on continuous improvement and well-being.

Use this prompt to explore your thoughts and feelings, and to set intentions for continuous improvement and personal growth, by heading over to the journal prompts for kaizen in chapter 26. Happy journaling!

七

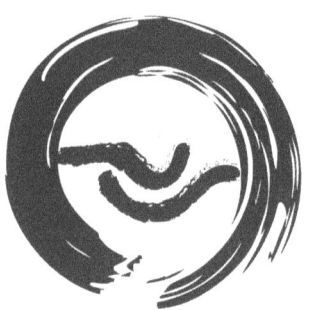

Shikata ga nai
Accept What Cannot Be Helped

CHAPTER 7

Shikata ga nai – Accept What Cannot Be Helped

In life, we are often confronted with situations that are beyond our control. Whether it's a sudden change in circumstances, an unexpected setback, or a challenge that seems insurmountable, we all face moments when things don't go as planned. In these times, we must remember the Japanese principle of *Shikata ga nai* 仕方がない, which translates to "it cannot be helped." This principle encourages us to accept that some things are simply beyond our control and that fighting against them is not productive.

While this might sound like a resignation to fate, *Shikata ga nai* is not about giving up or ignoring problems, it's about choosing to respond with grace, resilience, and a positive mindset. It's about recognizing when it's time to stop struggling and instead shift our energy toward moving forward in a healthier, more peaceful way.

1. **Meditate – Find Inner Peace Amidst Chaos**

Meditation is a powerful tool for cultivating peace within, especially during challenging times. By taking a moment to quiet your mind and focus on the present, you can reduce stress and anxiety. Meditation helps us disconnect from the noise of the world and tune into our inner wisdom. It teaches us to be in the moment and to let go of what we cannot control.

Try a simple breathing meditation: sit quietly, close your eyes, and focus on your breath. Inhale slowly through your nose, hold for a moment, and exhale through your mouth. With each breath, release tension and let go of your worries. More about meditation in chapter 15.

2. **Breathe Deeply – Activate Calmness**

Deep breathing is a quick and effective way to centre yourself. When life throws challenges your way, your body's natural response is often stress or anxiety, which can lead to shallow, rapid breathing. Deep breathing helps counteract this reaction by stimulating the parasympathetic nervous system, which induces a calm state.

Try the 4-7-8 method: inhale deeply for 4 seconds, hold your breath for 7 seconds, and exhale slowly for 8 seconds. Repeat this process for several rounds to bring your body into a relaxed state.

3. Immerse Yourself in Something Positive – Shift Your Focus

When things go wrong, it's easy to get stuck in negative thinking patterns. But *Shikata ga nai* reminds us to move forward, not stay stuck in frustration. One way to do this is by immersing yourself in something positive, whether it's listening to uplifting music, reading a motivational book, or watching an inspiring movie. This shift in focus helps you see life from a more positive perspective.

You can also engage in a hobby or activity that brings you joy, like painting, gardening, or playing an instrument. Immersing yourself in something that brings you happiness creates a mental space for healing.

4. Pick Yourself Up – Cultivate Resilience

Resilience is the ability to bounce back after adversity. *Shikata ga nai* teaches us to acknowledge our emotions, but not to dwell on them. When something goes wrong, it's okay to feel upset or disappointed but it's important to pick yourself up and move forward.

Start by acknowledging your feelings without judgment. Then, remind yourself that setbacks are part of the journey and not the end. Take small, actionable steps toward recovery, no matter how insignificant they may seem. Each step forward is progress.

5. Tune In – Listen to Your Inner Voice

Sometimes, accepting what cannot be helped requires us to listen to our intuition. In moments of uncertainty, our inner voice can provide guidance. Tune in to how you feel physically and emotionally. What is your body telling you? What does your intuition suggest?

When you take the time to listen to your inner voice, you gain clarity about the next steps you should take. Trust in yourself and your ability to make decisions that align with your well-being.

6. Always Be Learning – Turn Challenges into Lessons

One of the most valuable lessons we can learn from *Shikata ga nai* is that every experience, even the challenging ones, holds valuable wisdom. Instead of resisting or resenting difficult situations, try to view them as opportunities to learn and grow.

Ask yourself: What can I learn from this situation? How can I improve moving forward? When you embrace a mindset of constant learning, you begin to see challenges not as obstacles, but as opportunities for personal development.

7. Stop Comparing – Focus on Your Own Path

Comparison is often a trap that keeps us focused on what others are doing and away from what is right for us. *Shikata ga nai* encourages us to let go of the need to compare ourselves to others. Everyone has their own journey, and their path is not yours. Focus on your own progress and growth instead of measuring yourself against others.

Embrace your uniqueness and accept where you are in life. This acceptance fosters self-love and helps you stay focused on your own journey.

8. Tend to Your Own Garden – Nurture Yourself

Metaphorically, your life is like a garden. In order to flourish, you must tend to it with care and attention. This means taking care of your physical, mental, and emotional well-being. Nourish your body with healthy food, get adequate rest, and engage in activities that make you feel happy and fulfilled.

When you prioritize self-care and focus on nurturing yourself, you create the conditions for growth and well-being, regardless of external circumstances.

9. Look Into Healing – Explore Ways to Heal Yourself

Healing is a crucial part of accepting what cannot be helped. Whether through therapy, energy healing, journaling, nutrition, food supplements or physical self-care, it's important to find methods of healing that work for you. Healing helps you release the emotional weight of challenging situations and empowers you to move forward with a sense of peace. For ideas on Japanese healing methods, read chapter 16.

Explore different healing practices and choose the ones that resonate with you. Healing is not a destination, but an ongoing journey of self-acceptance and restoration.

10. **Change Your Perspective – Shift Your Viewpoint**

Sometimes, a simple shift in perspective can make all the difference. *Shikata ga nai* teaches us to accept situations as they are, but it also encourages us to find new ways to look at things. Instead of viewing a setback as a failure, try to see it as an opportunity for growth.

Ask yourself: How can I reframe this situation to see it in a more positive light? Changing your perspective can empower you to embrace challenges with a sense of curiosity and resilience.

11. **Forest Bathing – Connect with Nature**

Shikata ga nai also encourages us to reconnect with nature, as nature has an incredible way of helping us let go of stress and find peace. Forest bathing, or *Shinrin-yoku*, is a Japanese practice of immersing oneself in nature to benefit from its calming and healing effects.

Take a walk through a forest, park, or natural area. Allow the sights, sounds, and smells of nature to ground you. This practice can help you find perspective, clear your mind, and reduce stress.

12. **Hang Out with Supportive Friends – Build a Support System**

Lastly, one of the best ways to accept what cannot be helped is to surround yourself with people who offer encouragement and support. Having a strong social network of friends, family, or a community can help you navigate tough times with a sense of security and comfort.

Reach out to those who make you feel seen, heard, and understood. Let them remind you of your strength and ability to overcome challenges. Sometimes, just knowing you're not alone is all you need to accept and move forward.

Shikata ga nai is about embracing the inevitable uncertainties and challenges of life. It's about learning how to let go of what we cannot control and instead, focus on finding peace, healing, and acceptance in the face of adversity. By practicing meditation, nurturing our well-being, shifting our perspective, and surrounding ourselves with positivity, we can move through life's difficulties with grace and resilience.

Life doesn't always go as planned, but by accepting what cannot be helped, we free ourselves to focus on what we can change, and in doing so, we create space for greater peace, growth, and happiness.

This phrase shika ga nai, embodies a mindset of acceptance and resilience, which can support longevity in several ways:

1. **Stress Reduction:** By accepting situations that are beyond our control, "Shika ga nai" helps reduce stress and anxiety. Chronic stress is linked to numerous health issues, so managing stress effectively can contribute to a longer, healthier life.
2. **Emotional Resilience:** Embracing "Shika ga nai" fosters emotional resilience, allowing individuals to cope

better with life's challenges and setbacks. This resilience can enhance mental health and overall well-being.

3. **Focus on the Present:** The phrase encourages individuals to focus on the present moment rather than dwelling on past regrets or future uncertainties. Mindfulness and living in the present are associated with improved mental health and longevity.

4. **Adaptability:** "Shika ga nai" promotes adaptability and flexibility, encouraging individuals to adjust to changing circumstances. This adaptability can lead to better problem-solving and decision-making, supporting long-term health and success.

5. **Positive Outlook:** By accepting what cannot be changed, individuals can maintain a more positive outlook on life. Optimism and a positive attitude are linked to better health outcomes and increased longevity.

6. **Letting Go of Control:** Understanding that not everything is within our control allows individuals to focus their energy on what they can change. This focus can lead to more effective actions and healthier choices.

By adopting the mindset of "Shika ga nai," individuals can cultivate a sense of peace and acceptance, which can enhance their quality of life and contribute to longevity.

If you feel like heading over to the journal prompts for this chapter, then do so now and turn to chapter 26, otherwise, please make a note to return to journal and go deeper to feel that sense of peace and wholeness, completeness that enhances your longevity and quality of life.

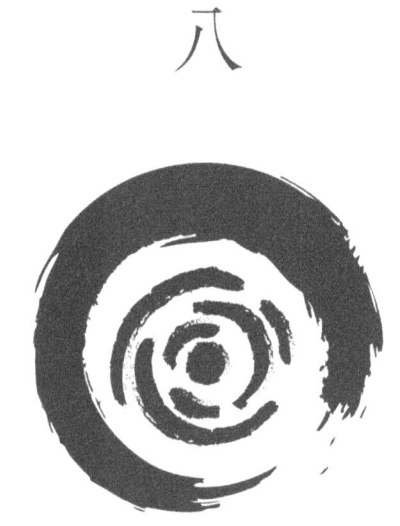

Yumaru
Care for Your Inner Circle

CHAPTER 8

Yumaru – Care for Your Inner Circle

In today's dynamic and ever-evolving environment, it's easy to forget the importance of the relationships that truly matter, the ones that nurture our growth and provide us with support and connection. *Yumaru* ゆまる, is a Japanese concept that emphasizes the importance of caring for your inner circle, those closest to you, the people who truly matter in your life. It encourages us to take a proactive approach to our relationships, to be there for others, and to embrace the power of community.

The idea behind *Yumaru* is simple: the health of your relationships is as vital as your physical and mental well-being. By investing in those relationships and showing up for the people you care about, you build a strong foundation of trust, love, and support. This chapter will explore how to nurture your inner circle and why it's essential for personal growth and fulfilment.

1. **Make a Commitment – Be All In**

Building strong relationships takes time and effort. To genuinely care for your inner circle, you must make a commitment to show up for them, whether it's in times of joy or hardship. This commitment means prioritizing the people who matter most in your life and being fully present for them.

Making a commitment is about consistency, it's not just about being there when it's convenient, but about staying committed to your relationships through thick and thin. When you are fully committed, you show the people in your life that you value them and are dedicated to maintaining the bond you share.

2. **Embrace Community – Strength in Togetherness**

Human beings are inherently social creatures, and we thrive in community. *Yumaru* teaches us that we are stronger together. Our inner circle can take many forms: family, friends, colleagues, or even a group of like-minded individuals. Embracing community means fostering a sense of belonging and recognizing the value of connection with others.

Find opportunities to engage with your community, whether it's joining a club, attending social events, or supporting a cause that matters to you. The more you connect, the more you create a web of support and trust that will sustain you throughout life's challenges.

3. Show – Don't Tell – Actions Speak Louder

It's easy to say, "I care" or "I'm here for you," but showing up for others in tangible ways is what truly matters. *Yumaru* encourages us to demonstrate care through our actions, not just words. Being thoughtful, helping with tasks, offering a listening ear, or simply showing kindness can make a world of difference.

Sometimes, it's not about grand gestures, it's about the little things: offering a hand when someone is struggling, checking in on a friend when they're going through a hard time, or being present during important moments. These actions reinforce your commitment to those you care about and strengthen your bonds.

4. Be Thoughtful – Consider Others' Needs

To truly care for your inner circle, you need to be considerate of the needs, feelings, and perspectives of those around you. Being thoughtful means noticing when someone needs support, understanding when they need space, and offering encouragement without expecting anything in return.

Taking the time to think about what will bring comfort or joy to someone else is a powerful way to build connection. Thoughtfulness is an expression of empathy; it shows that you are aware of others' experiences and are willing to step outside of your own needs to make someone else feel seen and supported.

5. Be Present – Give the Gift of Your Attention

In today's world of constant distractions, being fully present is a rare and precious gift. *Yumaru* teaches us to value the people in our lives by giving them our undivided attention. When you're with someone, put away your phone, focus on the conversation, and engage deeply. This shows respect for the relationship and communicates that the person is worthy of your time and energy.

Being present isn't just about physical presence, it's about emotional availability as well. Make sure you are truly listening when someone is speaking, not just waiting for your turn to talk. Be emotionally available for those you care about so that they feel heard and valued.

6. Share Yourself – Open Up to Others

Authenticity is at the core of *Yumaru*. To build meaningful relationships, it's important to be open and vulnerable with those you care about. Sharing yourself, your thoughts, dreams, fears, and joys which helps create deeper connections and fosters a sense of trust and understanding.

When you share your true self, you invite others to do the same. Vulnerability allows for greater emotional intimacy, and it helps strengthen the bonds of friendship and family. Don't be afraid to let your guard down and show the real you because it's the first step in creating more genuine and supportive relationships.

7. Offer Support – Be There When It Matters

Sometimes, the most important thing you can do for someone is offer your support. Whether it's emotional support during a tough time, physical help with a task, or words of encouragement, being there when someone needs you can have a profound impact.

Yumaru teaches us to actively look for ways to offer support without waiting for someone to ask. Whether it's offering a shoulder to cry on, helping out with a project, or providing a listening ear, your support can make all the difference in someone's life.

8. Don't Expect Anything in Return – Give Without Strings Attached

One of the most beautiful aspects of caring for your inner circle is the opportunity to give freely. *Yumaru* encourages us to offer our care and support without expecting anything in return. This doesn't mean being a martyr, but it does mean giving selflessly and out of love, rather than out of obligation or the desire for something in return.

When you care for others without expectations, you create a cycle of kindness that ripples outward. This strengthens relationships and fosters a culture of mutual respect and generosity.

9. Be Proactive – Anticipate Needs and Take Initiative

Proactivity is key to *Yumaru*. Don't wait for someone to ask for help or for an opportunity to connect, take the initiative. Check in with friends and family, offer assistance before it's needed, and create opportunities for bonding. Proactive care shows that you are invested in the wellbeing of those around you and that you value the relationship enough to take action.

By anticipating the needs of those in your inner circle and stepping in before it's asked, you show that you are deeply committed to the relationship and are always looking for ways to nurture it.

Caring for your inner circle is one of the most meaningful ways to nurture your well-being and foster a life of joy and fulfilment. *Yumaru* teaches us that strong relationships are built on commitment, thoughtful actions, and mutual support. When you embrace this principle, you not only strengthen the bonds with those closest to you, but you also cultivate a sense of community and belonging that enriches your life.

By making a commitment to care for your inner circle, being proactive in offering support, and giving without expecting anything in return, you create an environment where love, trust, and connection can flourish. Remember, the true essence of *Yumaru* is to give, share, and support, knowing that in caring for others, we also nurture ourselves.

The journal prompt to this chapter encourages you to go deeper with your thoughts and write some action points to put in place for some small increments of learning. Turn to chapter 26 for journal prompts for yumaru.

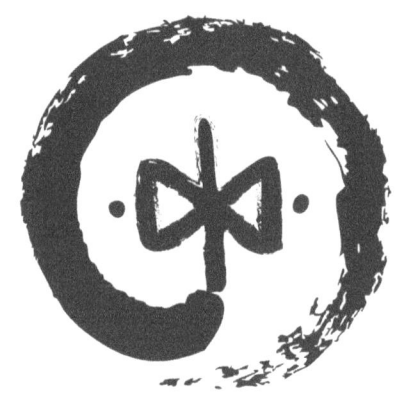

Kansha
Cultivate Sincere Gratitude

CHAPTER 9

Kansha – Cultivate Sincere Gratitude

Kansha 感謝, is the transformative power of gratitude. It not only brings joy to the giver but also radiates warmth to those around you. When you practice sincere gratitude, it's as though your smile extends from the heart, lighting up your life and the lives of others. But it's more than just an action, it's a mindset. Kansha teaches us to cultivate genuine appreciation for everything we have and everyone around us. By embracing gratitude, we shift our focus from what's lacking to what's abundant in our lives, opening our hearts to positivity and contentment.

Principles of Kansha – Cultivating Sincere Gratitude

1. **Your Smile Radiates from Your Heart!**

Gratitude is not just a fleeting feeling; it's a way of being. It's the warmth that emanates from your heart, creating an atmosphere of kindness, understanding, and joy. When you truly practice gratitude, it is reflected in your actions, your words, and even your smile. The power of a heartfelt smile is immeasurable; it not only brightens your day but can uplift the spirits of everyone you meet. Cultivating gratitude within yourself is the first step to becoming a radiant presence for those around you.

2. Cultivate Sincerity in Your Gratitude

Gratitude is not about checking off a list of things to be thankful for, it's about cultivating sincerity. Authenticity is key. When we express gratitude, it must come from the heart and not be a mere formality. Whether you're thanking someone for a small gesture or reflecting on the beauty of a sunrise, make sure your gratitude is genuine. By truly feeling gratitude, you bring an energy of sincerity that others can feel and appreciate. Gratitude that comes from the heart is deeply transformative, both for you and those around you.

Ways to Cultivate Sincere Gratitude:

- Be specific in your gratitude and acknowledge not just the actions but the intention behind them.
- Let your gratitude come from a place of deep awareness, rather than routine.
- Allow your gratitude to be felt in your body, plus express it through your actions, your tone, and your presence.

3. Practice Gratitude Every Day

Gratitude should be more than a once-in-a-while practice. It should be an integral part of your daily life. By incorporating gratitude into your everyday routine, you not only transform your mindset but also your experiences. Start each day with a moment of appreciation, perhaps you can make it a habit to write down three things you're grateful for each morning. Doing so primes your mind to look for the positive aspects of your life and fosters an attitude of abundance rather than scarcity.

Ideas for Practicing Gratitude Daily:

- Start a gratitude journal by writing down three things you're grateful for each day, no matter how big or small.
- Take a moment to express thanks before meals, during commutes, or when you wake up.
- Share gratitude with those around you like thanking a colleague for their help, or tell your partner how much they mean to you.
- Practice mindfulness to appreciate the present moment. Be conscious of the little things, like the warmth of the sun, the comfort of your bed, or the beauty of a flower.

4. The Ripple Effect of Gratitude

Gratitude is contagious. When you express appreciation, it creates a ripple effect that spreads positivity. One simple act of gratitude can brighten someone's day, which in turn might inspire them to do something kind for someone else. The cycle continues, creating an environment of care, respect, and kindness. Gratitude has the power to shift the atmosphere wherever it is present, whether it's in a family, a workplace, or a community.

·

How Gratitude Creates a Ripple Effect:

- When you express genuine thanks to someone, it boosts their mood and encourages them to share that joy with others.
- It fosters a culture of appreciation and kindness, which can positively affect both personal and professional environments.
- Acknowledging the small things helps to highlight the goodness around us, creating an upward cycle of positivity.

5. **Transforming Challenges through Gratitude**

Life is filled with both triumphs and challenges, and while it's easy to express gratitude when things are going well, it's the ability to find gratitude during difficult times that truly transforms us. Kansha teaches us that there is something to be grateful for in all experiences. Even in the face of hardship, we can choose to focus on the lessons, the strength gained, or the relationships that support us. Gratitude, in this sense, becomes a powerful tool for resilience and perspective.

Ways Gratitude Helps Us Through Challenges:

- Shifts focus from pain to growth, helping us to see obstacles as opportunities for learning.
- Reduces stress by encouraging a shift from a mindset of lack to one of abundance.
- Promotes emotional healing by allowing us to find silver linings, even in difficult situations.

6. **Gratitude for the Present Moment**

Often, we focus on what's coming next, what we're striving for or what we haven't yet achieved. While goals are important, true contentment comes from appreciating the present moment. Kansha encourages us to express gratitude for the now, whether it's the people in our lives, the work we're doing, or simply the breath we are taking. This mindfulness approach helps us to be fully present and cultivate a deeper sense of fulfilment.

Practices for Gratitude in the Present Moment:

- Practice mindfulness meditation to increase awareness of the present.
- Take regular moments to pause, breathe, and appreciate where you are, rather than rushing ahead.
- Focus on your senses and notice the sounds, sights, and textures around you and be thankful for the richness of life.

Gratitude isn't just an action; it's a way of being. When we cultivate sincere gratitude, it changes how we see the world and interact with others. It allows us to embrace both the good and the bad with a sense of appreciation, opening the door to deeper connection and inner peace. Gratitude becomes a mirror, reflecting all that is good, abundant, and meaningful in our lives. It empowers us to live with more joy, compassion, and purpose, while also inspiring those around us to do the same.

Gratitude can significantly contribute to longevity by fostering a positive mindset and promoting overall well-being. Here's how gratitude supports a longer, healthier life:

1. **Improves Mental Health:** Regularly practicing gratitude can reduce symptoms of depression and anxiety. A positive mental state is closely linked to better physical health and longevity.

2. **Enhances Emotional Resilience:** Gratitude helps individuals focus on the positive aspects of life, building emotional resilience. This resilience allows people to cope better with stress and adversity, which can enhance longevity.

3. **Strengthens Relationships:** Expressing gratitude can improve relationships by fostering feelings of connection and appreciation. Strong social ties are associated with longer life spans and better health outcomes.

4. **Reduces Stress:** Gratitude can lower stress levels by shifting focus from negative to positive experiences. Chronic stress is detrimental to health, so reducing stress can contribute to a longer life.

5. **Boosts Physical Health:** People who practice gratitude often report fewer physical symptoms, better sleep, and a stronger immune system. These factors all contribute to overall health and longevity.

6. **Encourages Healthy Behaviours:** Gratitude can motivate individuals to engage in healthier behaviours, such as regular exercise and balanced nutrition, which are essential for a long, healthy life.

7. **Promotes Mindfulness:** Practicing gratitude encourages mindfulness and being present in the moment. Mindfulness is associated with reduced stress and improved well-being, both of which support longevity.

By incorporating gratitude into daily life, individuals can enhance their mental, emotional, and physical health, ultimately contributing to a longer and more fulfilling life.

So, let your smile radiate from your heart, practice gratitude every day, and let it become a part of your way of living. Through gratitude, you will not only enrich your own life but the lives of everyone you encounter.

If you want to write your thoughts of gratitude or delve deeper into this chapter, turn to the journal prompts in chapter 26. I'm so grateful for you and getting this far into the book. Thank you so much, it means so much to me.

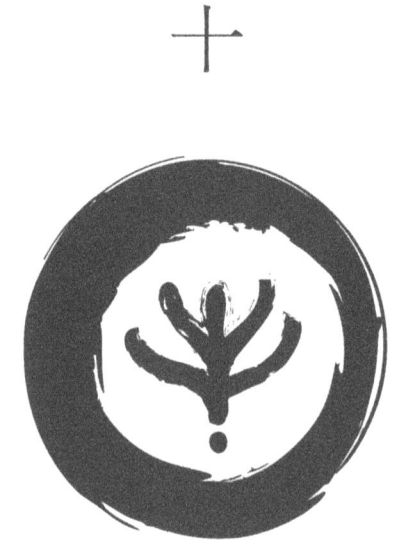

Osettai
Be of Service to Others

CHAPTER 10

Osettai – Be of Service to Others

The concept of Osettai お世話, is one that speaks to the heart of human connection. It is a Japanese principle that invites us to not just be present in the lives of others, but to actively contribute in ways that uplift, support, and add value to the world around us. The essence of Osettai is about selflessly offering our time, energy, and skills without expectation, knowing that true fulfilment comes from helping others.

In this chapter, we'll explore how you can adopt the mindset of service and apply it to your life in three profound ways: Sharing your talents, sharing your knowledge, and sharing your heart. Each of these approaches is vital in building stronger connections, nurturing personal growth, and contributing to a world that thrives on collective support.

1. Share Your Talents

Everyone has a unique set of talents, skills, and abilities. These are the gifts that make you, *you*. Whether you're an expert in something specific, have an artistic flair, or possess a gift for listening, your talents are your way to make a difference in the world.

To be of service to others through your talents, you must first recognize them. Often, we underestimate the value of what we can do, thinking that what comes easily to us is not extraordinary. But the truth is, your talents are exactly what the world needs. By sharing your strengths with others, you not only help them, but you also unlock your potential to create lasting change.

Practical Application:

- Volunteer your time to teach a skill you possess.
- Offer your expertise to someone in need of guidance.
- Use your talents to contribute to causes that align with your values.

2. **Share Your Knowledge**

Knowledge is one of the most valuable assets you can offer to others. It's not just about academic knowledge or professional expertise; it's also about life lessons, personal experiences, and the wisdom you've gathered over time. When you share what you know, you empower others to take informed actions, make better decisions, and grow.

However, sharing knowledge goes beyond simply giving information. It's about teaching, guiding, and mentoring. When you impart knowledge, you open doors to new possibilities, helping others overcome challenges they might face. The act of sharing what you know fosters a sense of collaboration, making the community or organization you're part of stronger and more resilient.

Practical Application:

- Mentor someone who can benefit from your expertise.
- Teach a class or workshop on a subject you're passionate about.
- Share a blog, article, or book that can help others grow.

3. **Share Your Heart**

The most powerful form of service is the one that comes from a place of genuine care and compassion. When you offer your heart to others, you give not only your time and energy, but also your empathy and understanding. It's the ability to be fully present in someone else's experience, offering support when it's needed most.

Sharing your heart involves listening deeply, offering a shoulder to lean on, or simply being there for someone without judgment. It's about creating an environment where people feel safe, valued, and understood. Your emotional investment in others has the power to heal wounds, provide comfort, and build strong, lasting relationships.

Practical Application:

- Take time to listen to someone who needs to talk.
- Offer emotional support to friends or colleagues going through tough times.
- Act with kindness and patience in all your interactions.

Why Osettai is Important in Your Life

Being of service to others through Osettai not only helps those around you, but it also enriches your own life. When you share your talents, knowledge, and heart, you experience a sense of fulfilment that cannot be gained through selfish pursuits. You discover the true joy of giving, not because you expect something in return, but because you know your actions make a difference.

Service strengthens communities, whether they're your family, workplace, or local neighbourhood. It fosters a sense of interconnectedness and compassion, making the world a better place, one small act of kindness at a time.

Osettai in Action

Here are a few ways to practice Osettai in your day-to-day life:

1. Volunteer your time and skills. Whether it's helping at a local shelter, tutoring someone, or offering your professional expertise for a worthy cause, giving your time can create ripples of positive change.
2. Be generous with your emotional support. A kind word, an open ear, or a gesture of encouragement can make all the difference in someone's day.
3. Mentor or guide others. Share your knowledge by mentoring someone who is just starting out in your field or offering career advice to someone in need.
4. Foster a culture of service in your work or family. Encourage those around you to be generous with their

talents and resources. Lead by example and create an environment where service is valued.

Incorporating Osettai into your life means understanding that we all have something valuable to offer. By sharing our talents, knowledge, and hearts with others, we contribute to the greater good and experience a deeper sense of purpose. True service doesn't require grand gestures, just consistent acts of kindness, support, and care.

As you continue your journey of growth, remember that service is not about doing everything for everyone, it's about doing what you can, where you are, and with what you have. Through Osettai, we create a world where the collective well-being of others matters just as much as our own, and we all rise together. This concept can contribute to longevity in several meaningful ways:

1. **Fosters Social Connections:** Engaging in osettai helps build strong social networks and a sense of community. Social connections are linked to better health outcomes and increased longevity, as they provide emotional support and reduce feelings of isolation.
2. **Enhances Emotional Well-being:** Acts of kindness and giving can boost emotional well-being by promoting feelings of happiness and fulfilment. Positive emotions are associated with improved mental health and a longer life.
3. **Reduces Stress:** Practicing osettai can reduce stress by shifting focus from personal worries to helping

others. Lower stress levels are beneficial for both mental and physical health, contributing to longevity.

4. **Promotes a Sense of Purpose:** Engaging in selfless acts provides a sense of purpose and meaning in life. Having a strong sense of purpose is linked to better health and longevity, as it motivates individuals to take care of themselves and others.

5. **Encourages a Positive Outlook:** Osettai encourages a positive outlook on life by emphasizing compassion and empathy. A positive mindset is associated with better health outcomes and increased life expectancy.

6. **Strengthens Community Resilience:** By promoting kindness and support within a community, osettai helps create a resilient environment where individuals can thrive and support each other, enhancing overall community health and longevity.

Incorporating the spirit of osettai into daily life can lead to a more connected, compassionate, and fulfilling existence, ultimately supporting a longer and healthier life.

Take a moment to reflect and capture your thoughts on the concept of osettai in your journal in chapter 26.

十一

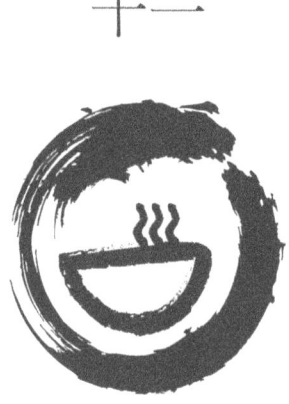

Chado
The Pleasures of Matcha and the Japanese Tea Culture

CHAPTER 11

Chado - The Pleasures of Matcha and the Japanese Tea Culture

My first encounter with a traditional Japanese tea ceremony was a moment of complete wonder, leaving me both captivated and intrigued. It was in this moment that my fascination with the art of the Japanese tea ceremony truly began.

During my ten years in Japan, I fully immersed myself in this beautiful tradition, taking tea ceremony lessons, donning kimonos, learning about tea utensils, and even taking pottery classes in the historic town of Nara, where I lived from 1992 to 2001. My goal was to create my very own tea ceremony bowl, which I still cherish and use today.

One of the aspects of Japanese culture that I truly admire is the sense of hospitality. Whether at someone's home, an office, or a traditional family-run ryokan (Japanese B&B), visitors are always warmly welcomed with a cup of freshly brewed green tea. This practice, deeply ingrained in Japanese society, is a reflection of the country's warm and respectful approach to both guests and life in general.

The history of the tea ceremony, known as *chado* 茶道, dates back to the 12th century. Tea was first introduced to Japan from China, and it is widely documented that the Zen monk Eisai (1141–1215) wrote *Kissa Yojoku* ("Drinking Tea for Health"), which highlighted the health benefits of tea, particularly matcha. Monks would drink tea to remain alert during long hours of meditation, and eventually, the practice spread from the temples to society at large. While the tea ceremony began as a spiritual ritual, in modern-day Japan, it has evolved into a cultural and social event that embodies both tradition and mindfulness.

Tea gardens and tea houses in Japan are designed with careful attention to detail, often built from wood and adorned with tatami straw flooring, delicate painted artwork, and minimalist furnishings. Each ceremony utilizes a set of specific utensils to enhance the experience, such as hanging scrolls, a kettle, water jar, flower container, tea bowl, tea scoop, tea caddy, incense, a whisk, and of course, matcha green tea. Additionally, a specialty sweet is often served to complement the tea, providing a harmonious balance to the overall experience.

Whenever I visit Japan, I make it a point to journey to Uji, a town renowned for its incredible matcha tea. Nestled in the picturesque Kyoto Prefecture, Uji is celebrated as the heart of Japan's matcha culture, offering an authentic and immersive experience for tea enthusiasts.

In Uji, the air is filled with the rich aroma of freshly ground matcha, and the landscape is dotted with lush tea fields that stretch as far as the eye can see. The town is home to some of the oldest and most revered tea houses, where skilled artisans meticulously prepare matcha using time-honoured techniques.

Each visit to Uji is an opportunity to savour the delicate, earthy flavours of matcha in its purest form, whether enjoyed in a traditional tea ceremony or as part of innovative culinary creations. Beyond the tea, Uji offers a serene escape with its historic temples, scenic riverside walks, and a deep sense of tranquility that invites reflection and rejuvenation.

Uji is not just a destination; it's a celebration of matcha's rich heritage and a testament to the artistry and dedication that goes into every cup.

The beauty and flow of the tea ceremony are both relaxing and deeply moving. While the formalities may seem rigid, each step is performed with grace, like a dance that has been perfected over time. I must admit, my first taste of matcha was somewhat unfamiliar and peculiar, but as I participated in more tea ceremonies with friends and colleagues, my appreciation for the ceremony and its significance deepened.

If you're seeking an authentic cultural experience, I highly recommend visiting Japan. The seamless blend of ancient traditions and modern living is evident throughout the country, particularly in the tea ceremony culture. In major department stores, you'll find entire aisles dedicated to matcha products, confections, and beautiful tea utensils, a testament to the continued vibrancy of this tradition. Japan is truly a destination that offers something profound for those who seek it.

I feel incredibly honoured to have had the opportunity to participate in such a timeless tradition. Even now, in my modern home in Poole, Dorset, England, I display my tea ceremony utensils with great pride, a constant reminder of the serene beauty and wisdom that this practice imparts.

Hosting Your Own Matcha Tea Ceremony at Home

To bring a piece of this beautiful tradition into your home, here's a simple guide to hosting your own matcha tea ceremony:

1. Gather Supplies:

   - Tea bowl (*chawan*)
   - Tea scoop (*chashaku*)
   - Tea whisk (*chasen*)
   - Tea caddy (*natsume*)

2. Prepare the Tea Bowl:

   - Begin by warming the tea bowl. Pour hot water into the bowl and swirl gently to ensure its warmed evenly.

3. Boil Water:

   - Boil water and allow it to cool slightly to the appropriate temperature for matcha ideally around 160–170°F (70–80°C).

4. Sift Matcha Powder:

   - Sift the matcha powder into the tea bowl to prevent any lumps, ensuring a smooth consistency.

5. Mix Water and Matcha:

- Pour the cooled water into the tea bowl with the sifted matcha powder. Prepare to mix the two together.

6. Whisk the Mixture:

- Use the tea whisk (*chasen*) to whisk the mixture. Do this briskly in a zig-zag motion until the matcha becomes frothy and vibrant green.

7. Serve and Enjoy:

- Once the matcha is ready, serve it to your guests, allowing everyone to share in the experience of mindfulness, connection, and respect.

Remember, a tea ceremony is not just about the tea itself, it's a chance to slow down, find peace, and escape the hustle and bustle of daily life. By taking the time to appreciate each step of the process, you can enjoy a moment of serenity, leaving your worries outside the tearoom.

Enjoy the calming, nourishing ritual of matcha tea, and let it guide you toward greater presence and tranquility in your life.

Green tea is renowned for its numerous health benefits, many of which contribute to longevity. Here are some key benefits:

1. **Rich in Antioxidants:** Green tea is packed with polyphenols, particularly catechins like EGCG, which are powerful antioxidants. These compounds help

combat oxidative stress and reduce the risk of chronic diseases.

2. **Improves Brain Function:** The caffeine and L-theanine in green tea can enhance brain function, improving mood, vigilance, reaction time, and memory. Regular consumption may also protect against neurodegenerative diseases like Alzheimer's and Parkinson's.

3. **Supports Heart Health:** Green tea is linked to improved heart health by lowering LDL cholesterol and triglycerides, reducing blood pressure, and improving blood vessel function. These factors collectively reduce the risk of cardiovascular diseases.

4. **Aids Weight Management:** Green tea can boost metabolic rate and increase fat burning, aiding in weight management. Maintaining a healthy weight is crucial for longevity.

5. **Reduces Cancer Risk:** The antioxidants in green tea may lower the risk of certain cancers, including breast, prostate, and colorectal cancers, by protecting cells from DNA damage.

6. **Enhances Longevity:** Regular consumption of green tea is associated with a lower risk of death from all causes, particularly cardiovascular disease, contributing to a longer life.

7. **Supports Immune Function:** The catechins in green tea have antibacterial and antiviral properties that can enhance immune function and protect against infections.

8. **Promotes Healthy Aging:** The anti-inflammatory properties of green tea help reduce inflammation, a key factor in aging and age-related diseases.

Incorporating green tea into your daily routine can be a simple yet effective way to support overall health and longevity.

Seize the opportunity to enhance your well-being by jotting down a commitment in your journal to purchase some high-quality green tea, whether it's loose leaf or matcha. By incorporating this ancient elixir into your daily routine, you can unlock a myriad of health benefits.

Green tea, with its rich antioxidant profile, not only invigorates the senses but also supports your journey towards a healthier lifestyle. Whether you choose the delicate, earthy notes of loose leaf or the vibrant, ceremonial experience of matcha, integrating green tea into your daily regimen can lead to improved mental clarity, enhanced metabolism, and a fortified immune system.

Make this small yet impactful change today and experience the rejuvenating effects that green tea can bring to your life. Your future self will thank you for this mindful addition to your wellness routine.

You can journal about green tea, the ceremony, the health benefits and how taking a few minutes to just drink a cup of green tea gives you time to recalibrate your thoughts. Head over to chapter 26 for more journal prompts.

十二

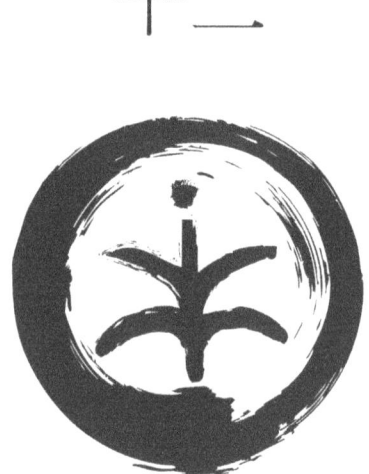

Ikebana
The Art of Flower Arranging

CHAPTER 12

Ikebana - The Art of Flower Arranging

One of the most beautiful and calming practices I had the privilege of experiencing during my time in Japan was the art of Ikebana, or Japanese flower arranging. I've always had a love for nature and the elegance of flowers, and it was such a joy to bring a little piece of nature into my home through floral designs.

Ikebana, also known as *kadō* 華道 (the way of flowers), is far more than simply arranging flowers in a vase. It is a meditative and artistic practice that seeks to bring out the soul of the flowers, branches, leaves, and stems. This ancient art form isn't just about placing flowers for decoration, it's about creating harmony, balance, and a deeper connection to nature and oneself.

The word "Ikebana" translates to "making flowers come alive," which beautifully captures the essence of this art. Each arrangement is a living, breathing expression of the natural world. Ikebana practitioners carefully consider the lines, colours, mass, form, and movement of each element, as well as the space around them, to create a balance between the floral design and its surroundings. The arrangement is meant to represent not only the beauty of nature but also the imperfection and transience of life, which is such an important concept in Japanese culture.

Ikebana has roots that stretch back over 600 years to the time of the early Buddhist temples, where offerings of flowers were made to the gods. It evolved over the centuries into the refined art form we recognize today. The practice reflects the Japanese appreciation for the fleeting beauty of nature, where flowers bloom, and then gracefully fade away, reminding us to embrace the present moment.

During my time in Japan, I took part in Ikebana lessons, and I found it to be a wonderful way to slow down and appreciate the beauty around me. The process itself is meditative. Each flower, stem, and leaf are treated with mindfulness and care. What I love most about Ikebana is that, unlike Western-style floral arrangements, it doesn't aim to be lush or over-the-top. Instead, it focuses on simplicity, space, and the natural flow of the materials used. It's about creating beauty through restraint, using just a few elements to convey meaning and emotion.

Getting Started with Ikebana

Ikebana is surprisingly accessible, and it doesn't require fancy materials or a lot of experience to begin. In fact, you can start with what you already have around you! Here's how you can begin your own Ikebana practice at home:

1. Gather Basic Tools
   You don't need to invest in expensive tools to start. A basic set of scissors, a simple vase or container, and floral foam (or a similar holder) are all you need to get started. You can even improvise with household items, as the real beauty of Ikebana lies in your creativity and connection to nature.

2. Start with Simple Arrangements
   Begin with easy-to-find flowers and branches. You don't have to use exotic blooms—local flowers and greenery work just as well. Focus on understanding the basic principles: how the flowers' shapes, colours, and textures interact. Pay attention to their individual beauty and let that inspire your design.

3. Observe Nature
   One of the best ways to understand Ikebana is by observing the world around you. Take walks in nature, whether it's a park, garden, or even your backyard. Look at how plants grow, how branches bend, and how flowers form in the wild. Pay attention to the natural asymmetry and the way plants are shaped by their environment. This will help you embrace the concept of "perfect imperfection" that is central to Ikebana.

4. Experiment with Shapes and Proportions
   Ikebana is all about balance, and this can be tricky at first. Experiment with different proportions and placements. For example, try using tall, sweeping lines contrasted with shorter, more compact elements. Play with the idea of "empty space" in the arrangement, this space is just as important as the flowers themselves and allows the arrangement to breathe.

5. Embrace Imperfections
   Don't worry about making your arrangements "perfect."
   In fact, imperfection is a key element in Ikebana. Nature
   itself is imperfect, and this is reflected in the art. Allow
   your arrangements to flow naturally and don't be afraid
   to make mistakes. The process of creation is just as
   important as the final result.

Ikebana is much more than a decorative practice; it is an opportunity to slow down, reflect, and connect with the present moment. As you work with flowers, you'll likely find yourself meditating on the fragility of life and the beauty that surrounds us. And as you begin to incorporate more Ikebana into your life, you might notice a sense of calmness and balance that extends beyond your floral creations into other areas of your life.

The Philosophy of Ikebana

At the heart of Ikebana is the idea that the flowers, stems, and leaves are all living beings, and they should be treated with the same respect that you would show to any other living creature. Each element is considered carefully, and the arrangement is a reflection of nature's beauty and impermanence.

There are many styles of Ikebana, ranging from formal and symmetrical to informal and freeform. But no matter which style you choose, the essence of the practice remains the same: it's about creating balance and harmony between nature, the artist, and the viewer. It's an opportunity to connect with your inner self, to appreciate the simple beauty of nature, and to create something that reflects both your emotions and the world around you.

So, whether you're looking to decorate your home with beauty or simply find a new way to connect with nature, I highly encourage you to try Ikebana. It is a practice that nurtures both the body and the soul, and it is something that can enrich your life in unexpected ways.

As you begin this journey, remember there are no "mistakes" in Ikebana. The flowers will guide you, and the process will reveal its own unique beauty. Enjoy the tranquility and creativity that comes with this peaceful and meaningful art form.

Ikebana also offers several benefits that can contribute to longevity and overall well-being:

1. **Stress Reduction:** Engaging in ikebana requires focus and mindfulness, which can help reduce stress and promote relaxation. Lower stress levels are linked to improved heart health and a stronger immune system, both of which are important for longevity.

2. **Enhances Mindfulness:** The practice of arranging flowers encourages mindfulness and being present in the moment. This can lead to a greater sense of peace and mental clarity, reducing anxiety and enhancing emotional wellbeing.

3. **Boosts Creativity:** Ikebana is a creative outlet that allows individuals to express themselves artistically. Engaging in creative activities is associated with

improved cognitive function and can help keep the mind sharp as we age.

4. **Promotes Connection with Nature:** Ikebana fosters a deep appreciation for nature and its beauty. This connection with nature can enhance mood and provide a sense of tranquility, contributing to overall mental health.

5. **Encourages Patience and Discipline:** The meticulous nature of ikebana requires patience and discipline, qualities that can be beneficial in other areas of life. Developing these traits can lead to better decision-making and a more balanced lifestyle.

6. **Social Interaction:** Participating in ikebana classes or groups provides opportunities for social interaction, which is crucial for emotional health and longevity. Building and maintaining social connections can reduce feelings of loneliness and increase life satisfaction.

By incorporating ikebana into your life, you can enjoy these holistic benefits that support both mental and physical health, ultimately contributing to a longer and more fulfilling life.

Head over to the journal prompt for ikebana and document your experience, noting any insights or feelings of peace and creativity that emerge. How might you incorporate ikebana into your regular routine to enhance your well-being and connection with nature?

Use this prompt to explore the deeper impact of ikebana on your life and how it can contribute to your overall sense of well-being and longevity, so head over to chapter 26 for more thought-provoking journal prompts.

十三

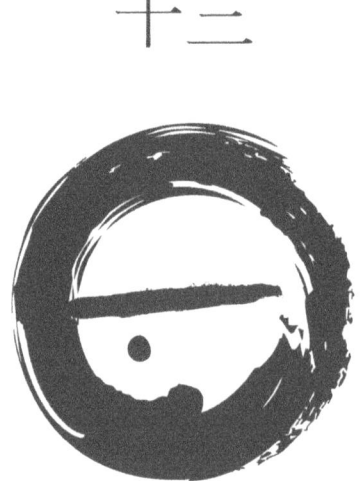

Kanso
Embracing Simplicity Through Decluttering

CHAPTER 13

Kanso – Embracing Simplicity Through Decluttering

The Japanese Art of Simplicity: Kanso

In Japanese culture, the concept of *Kanso* (簡素) holds profound significance, particularly when applied to the art of living and organizing one's home. Translated simply as "simplicity" or "minimalism," *Kanso* encourages a life that is uncluttered, straightforward, and free from excess. The roots of *Kanso* extend far beyond the mere removal of unnecessary possessions; it is about creating an environment that fosters clarity, peace, and balance.

Decluttering through the lens of *Kanso* isn't just about creating a visually clean or empty space. It's about intentionally choosing what to keep and what to release, with the ultimate goal of creating a harmonious and calming environment. This is rooted in the belief that our external surroundings deeply impact our inner state. A cluttered space often results in a cluttered mind, while a well-curated environment can promote a sense of tranquility and focus.

The Science Behind Decluttering and Its Benefits

There is growing scientific evidence to support the benefits of decluttering, both for our mental and physical health. Clutter, in its many forms, can act as a source of stress. In fact, studies show that disorganized spaces can increase cortisol levels, the body's primary stress hormone, leading to feelings of anxiety and overwhelm.

1. Mental Health: Studies show that clutter can contribute to feelings of anxiety, stress, and even depression. The constant visual reminders of disorganization can lead to a heightened sense of overwhelm, making it difficult to focus on tasks or even relax at home. According to a study conducted at the University of California, Los Angeles (UCLA), cluttered environments contribute to increased stress and a feeling of being "out of control." This ties into the concept of *Kanso*, so when we eliminate clutter, we create space for mental clarity and a sense of ease. A minimalist, organized environment can help reduce stress, promote focus, and encourage a sense of peace.

2. Productivity and Focus: Another benefit of decluttering is its positive effect on productivity. Research from Princeton University's Neuroscience Institute found that clutter in the home or workspace can reduce our ability to focus. When our environment is filled with excess, our brains are forced to divide attention between tasks and the clutter. This constant switching reduces efficiency and mental clarity. *Kanso* offers the opposite approach which shows us that a clean,

organized environment that encourages uninterrupted focus and helps to improve decision-making.

3. The Impact on Sleep: Clutter can also interfere with our quality of sleep. A study from the Sleep Health Foundation found that cluttered or messy bedrooms can negatively affect the quality of sleep. When we are surrounded by disorganization, it sends a signal to our brains that we are not in control of our environment, which can make it harder to relax. Adopting *Kanso* in our bedrooms and living spaces promotes a peaceful and orderly environment, which supports relaxation and leads to better sleep.

The Principles of *Kanso* in Daily Life

To truly embrace *Kanso*, one must begin to view possessions with a discerning eye. *Kanso* is not about getting rid of everything, but rather about retaining only what serves a purpose or brings joy. Here are a few principles of *Kanso* that can help guide your decluttering process:

1. Value Function Over Excess: When it comes to both objects and activities in our lives, it's important to consider whether they truly add value. Japanese culture often focuses on functionality and utility. Each item in your home should serve a clear purpose, either functionally or aesthetically. As you begin to declutter, ask yourself: Does this item serve a purpose? Does it bring me joy? Is it useful, or is it just taking up space?

2. Create Space for Peace: A key part of *Kanso* is the notion of "creating space", not just physical space,

but mental space as well. By removing unnecessary clutter, you can cultivate an environment that promotes relaxation and a sense of calm. This is reflected in the Japanese concept of *ma* (間), which refers to the space between things. It's not the objects themselves, but the spaces between them that contribute to harmony. Embrace the empty spaces in your home; they allow for ease and air, giving your surroundings room to breathe.

3. Curate, Don't Accumulate: Modern consumer culture often encourages us to accumulate more, like more clothes, more gadgets, more furniture. However, *Kanso* teaches us the importance of curation over accumulation. Take time to carefully choose and maintain only the things that enhance your life or hold deep personal value. Think of your home as a gallery, where each item is a purposeful addition to the overall harmony.

4. Tidy Regularly: Decluttering is not a one-time activity, but a practice that must be integrated into daily life. The Japanese are famous for their habitual cleaning practices, such as *osoji* (大掃除), the annual deep cleaning of homes. In daily life, tidying up becomes a ritual, not a burden. Regularly assess your surroundings and remove items that are no longer needed, keeping only those that contribute to the harmony of your space. This daily attention fosters a sense of responsibility and mindfulness.

5. Appreciate What You Have: The act of *Kanso* also encourages us to appreciate the simple and essential aspects of life. By removing distractions and excess, we become more attuned to the things that truly matter.

Whether it's a single flower vase on the table, a well-loved book, or a piece of artwork, *Kanso* teaches us to deeply appreciate the few items that bring us joy and meaning.

The Practical Steps to Embrace *Kanso* in Your Home

1. Start Small: If you're new to decluttering, start with one area of your home. It could be a shelf, a closet, or even your workspace. Tackle it with a clear intention: only keep what serves a purpose and get rid of anything that no longer aligns with your current lifestyle.

2. Let Go of Sentimental Clutter: Sentimental items can be the hardest to part with, but they can also hold us back from embracing *Kanso*. Take time to evaluate each item. If it no longer brings you joy or serves a purpose, let it go with gratitude for the memories it has provided. You can always take a photo to remember it by.

3. Consider Your Environment: Look at how your furniture and belongings are arranged. Is there a flow that promotes ease and relaxation, or is the space cramped and chaotic? Consider the energy you want to create in each room and how your possessions either support or hinder that.

4. Mindful Maintenance: Once you've decluttered, maintain the simplicity. Each time you acquire something new, ask yourself whether it truly fits with your values and serves a purpose in your life. *Kanso* is a continual process of curating your environment with intention.

Final note: The Power of Simplicity

By embracing *Kanso*, we are not just decluttering our homes, we are also creating a mindset that values simplicity, purpose, and mindfulness. In a world that often encourages excess and accumulation, the art of *Kanso* reminds us that less is often more. The science shows that a simple, decluttered environment reduces stress, increases focus, and promotes overall wellbeing. By bringing the principles of *Kanso* into your home, you invite a sense of peace and balance that can have a profound impact on both your physical space and your mental health.

Document your journey, noting any changes in your mood, energy levels, or sense of peace. How can embracing kanso as a regular practice enhance your overall wellness and contribute to a longer, more fulfilling life? Reflect on the impact of simplicity and intentional living on your path to longevity.

Use this journal prompt to delve deeper into the practice of kanso and its potential to enrich your life by fostering a serene and balanced environment. Head over to chapter 26 for more journal prompts.

十四

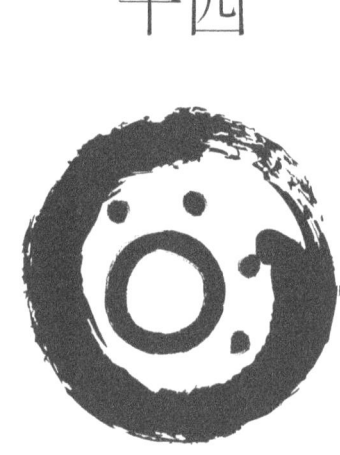

Ikigai
The Japanese Secret to a Fulfilling Life

CHAPTER 14

Ikigai – The Japanese Secret to a Fulfilling Life

Ikigai is a concept that has gained significant attention in recent years, both in Japan and around the world. It is a simple yet profound idea that translates roughly to "a reason for being" or "a reason to wake up in the morning." It refers to the intersection of four essential elements of life:

1. What you love (your passion)
2. What you are good at (your vocation)
3. What the world needs (your mission)
4. What you can be paid for (your profession)

When these elements align, you are said to have found your *ikigai*, a fulfilling purpose that not only drives you but also nourishes your mind, body, and soul. But it's not just a philosophical or emotional concept; science has started to back up the incredible health benefits of having *ikigai*.

The Science Behind Ikigai

In Japan, *ikigai* 生き甲斐, is considered a cornerstone of wellbeing. The Blue Zones, regions known for having the longest-lived people, are home to those who have found their *ikigai*, particularly in Okinawa, where it has been cited as a key factor in the longevity of its residents. Let's explore some of the science behind why having a strong sense of purpose is so beneficial for your health.

1. **Purpose and Longevity**

Research has shown that having a sense of purpose is linked to a longer, healthier life. A study published in *Psychological Science* found that individuals with a clear sense of purpose were significantly less likely to experience a decline in their physical health over time. The study found that purpose-driven individuals had lower levels of inflammation, better cardiovascular health, and fewer chronic conditions.

In Okinawa, Japan, where people live the longest in the world, the residents often attribute their longevity to having *ikigai*, a reason to live and something that keeps them active and engaged well into their 100s. It's not just about physical health; purpose also keeps them mentally active and emotionally fulfilled.

2. **Mental Health and Wellbeing**

Having a sense of purpose can profoundly affect mental health. A study by researchers at the University of California found that having a sense of purpose could lower the risk of depression and anxiety. The researchers found that people with a strong sense of purpose tended to have better coping mechanisms and were more resilient in the face of adversity.

In fact, individuals who are actively pursuing their *ikigai* tend to experience a higher level of happiness and life satisfaction. This sense of fulfilment is associated with increased levels of dopamine, the neurotransmitter responsible for feelings of pleasure and reward. The more aligned you are with your *ikigai*, the more dopamine your brain produces, reinforcing a sense of well-being.

3. Improved Sleep and Stress Reduction

People who have a clear sense of purpose are also likely to experience better sleep and lower stress levels. One study conducted by the National Institute of Aging found that individuals who reported having a purpose in life had better sleep quality and were less likely to experience sleep disturbances. This is because purpose can reduce cortisol, the stress hormone, and activate the parasympathetic nervous system, which promotes relaxation and rest.

Additionally, the sense of being engaged in something meaningful allows individuals to maintain a sense of calm even during stressful situations. In the practice of *ikigai*, the focus is on living authentically and with intention, which naturally reduces anxiety and promotes a more balanced state of mind.

4. Healthier Habits and Selfcare

People who are connected to their *ikigai* are more likely to take care of their health. They are more likely to eat nutritious food, exercise regularly, and avoid unhealthy habits. Studies have shown that individuals who find meaning and purpose in their lives tend to engage in more positive health behaviours.

In Okinawa, for instance, people have a saying: *Hara Hachi Bu*, which means "eat until you are 80% full." This principle, tied to their sense of purpose, encourages mindfulness around food and consumption, contributing to better digestion and weight management. They also engage in physical activities like walking, gardening, or participating in community activities, and activities that are tied to their *ikigai* and contribute to both their physical and mental wellbeing.

5. Social Connections and Community

At its core, *ikigai* is not just about individual fulfilment but also about connecting with others. People with a strong sense of purpose often have stronger social ties, and these connections are vital for longevity. A study published in *JAMA Psychiatry* found that having strong social bonds can reduce the risk of premature death and improve mental health.

In Japan, community plays a significant role in one's *ikigai*. People who are deeply embedded in their communities feel a sense of responsibility and connection, which contributes to both their mental health and longevity. The Okinawans, in particular, practice the concept of '*moai*', a form of social group that provides both emotional and financial support throughout life. These deep social connections create a support system that fosters resilience and wellbeing.

How to Find Your Ikigai

Finding your *ikigai* is a personal journey that involves deep introspection. While the process can take time, here are some steps you can take to begin uncovering your own *ikigai*.

1. Reflect on What You Love

What activities make you feel alive and energized? What brings you joy and fulfilment? Reflect on what you naturally gravitate toward and the passions that light you up.

2. Identify Your Strengths

What are you good at? What skills or talents do you possess? Understanding what you are naturally good at can help guide you toward your *ikigai*, as it often lies at the intersection of your talents and passions.

3. Consider What the World Needs

What problems or challenges in the world resonate with you? What needs can you fulfil through your skills and passions? This step connects you to the greater purpose of your *ikigai*, as it often involves contributing to something bigger than yourself.

4. Think About How You Can Be Rewarded

Finally, consider how you can be compensated for pursuing your *ikigai*. This doesn't always mean financial compensation, it can also refer to emotional or spiritual rewards. Reflect on how your purpose can bring balance to your life and sustain you.

Ikigai is not just a philosophy; it's a powerful, life-affirming practice that is backed by science. The concept encourages us to live with intention, to align our actions with our passions, and to serve a purpose that nurtures both ourselves and others. By embracing *ikigai*, we not only enrich our lives but also cultivate a healthier, more fulfilling existence and one that leads to greater longevity, improved mental health, and deeper social connections.

Embrace your *ikigai* and let it guide you on a journey to living a life that is truly meaningful.

Here's a journal prompt to help you explore and discover your ikigai:

Take a moment to reflect on the four key elements of ikigai: what you love, what you are good at, what the world needs, and what you can be paid for. Begin by listing activities or interests that bring you joy and fulfilment. What are the things you are passionate about, and why do they resonate with you?

Next, consider your skills and strengths. What are you naturally good at, and how have these abilities shaped your life? Reflect on how these skills can be used to address the needs of the world around you. What problems or challenges do you feel drawn to solve, and how can your unique talents contribute to making a positive impact?

Finally, explore opportunities where your passions and skills intersect with potential income. What services or products can you offer that align with your core values and provide value to others?

As you journal, consider how these elements come together to form your ikigai. How does this discovery influence your sense of purpose and direction in life? Reflect on any insights or realizations that emerge and consider how you can incorporate your ikigai into your daily life to create a more fulfilling and meaningful existence.

Use this prompt to delve deeper into your personal journey towards finding and living your ikigai. There's more journal prompts on ikigai in chapter 26.

十五

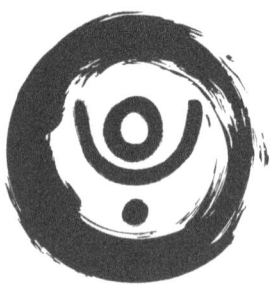

Meiso
Japanese Styles of Meditation and the Science of Stillness

CHAPTER 15

Meiso - Japanese Styles of Meditation and the Science of Stillness

One of the most powerful gifts I took from my time in Japan was the quiet discipline of meditation, Meiso 瞑想, which translates to 'closed-eye contemplation'. Japan has a long and rich tradition of contemplative practices, rooted in Zen Buddhism and Shintoism, that emphasize inner peace, awareness, and the deep connection between nature and the self.

Meditation in Japan isn't just a wellness trend, it is embedded in the culture, from the quiet rituals of tea ceremonies to the mindful raking of Zen gardens. Let's explore the unique Japanese meditation styles and what science tells us about their value

Popular Japanese Meditation Styles

1. Zazen (Seated Meditation)

   - Zazen, the core practice of Zen Buddhism, translates to "seated meditation."
   - Practiced in silence, often in a cross-legged position, Zazen encourages attention to the breath and the posture, allowing thoughts to come and go without attachment.
   - The purpose is not to "empty the mind," but to observe it, cultivate awareness, and access clarity and calm.

2. Kinhin (Walking Meditation)

   - Often practiced between long sessions of Zazen, Kinhin involves slow, deliberate walking while maintaining meditative focus.
   - Practitioners focus on the sensation of movement and the breath, anchoring awareness to the present moment.

3. Shikantaza ("Just Sitting")

   - A more advanced form of Zazen practiced mainly in the Soto Zen tradition.
   - Unlike other styles that focus on breath or mantras, Shikantaza involves no specific object of meditation, just awareness of *being*.
   - It teaches you to observe life as it is, without resistance or judgment.

4. Misogi (Shinto Purification Meditation)

- A Shinto practice of cleansing the body, mind, and spirit, often involving ritualistic movements, breathwork, or exposure to cold water (like waterfalls or rivers).
- It's about releasing negativity and re-centring within the rhythms of nature.

The Science Behind Meditation

Research on meditation, including styles like Zazen, shows significant health and cognitive benefits:

Stress Reduction

- Meditation reduces cortisol, the primary stress hormone, improving overall wellbeing.
- It activates the parasympathetic nervous system, which is responsible for "rest and digest" functions.

Brain Health

- MRI studies show that regular meditators have increased grey matter in areas linked to memory, learning, and emotional regulation.
- Meditation helps strengthen the prefrontal cortex, associated with focus and decision-making.

Emotional Regulation

- Regular meditation improves mood and reduces symptoms of anxiety and depression.

- It increases self-awareness and compassion, both for oneself and others.

Improved Sleep and Relaxation

- Meditative practices calm the mind and body, making it easier to fall and stay asleep.
- Techniques like mindful breathing activate the vagus nerve, promoting a state of deep relaxation.

Why Consistency Matters

In Japan, meditation is not seen as a one-off practice, it's a lifelong companion. Even just 5 to 10 minutes a day can attribute to noticeable improvements in mental clarity, patience, and overall energy.

The minimalist nature of Zazen mirrors the aesthetic of Kanso, no frills, just presence. That's the beauty of Japanese meditation: its simplicity makes it accessible, yet its depth keeps you learning for a lifetime.

How to Begin a Japanese-Inspired Meditation Practice

1. Create a quiet space – A cushion on the floor, a candle, or a small natural object can help centre your focus.
2. Sit comfortably – Cross-legged or on a chair with your spine straight.
3. Focus on your breath – Inhale through the nose, exhale slowly. Let thoughts pass without judgment.
4. Try a short Kinhin walk – Move slowly, coordinating each step with your breath.

5. Repeat daily – Even five minutes is a powerful place to start.

Meditation in Japan is not about perfection, it's about presence. It teaches us to stop grasping and just be. In a world that constantly asks us to do more, Japanese meditation offers a gentle invitation to simply be.

Meditation has been widely studied for its potential benefits on longevity and overall well-being. Here's a look at the correlation and science behind how meditation can contribute to a longer, healthier life:

1. **Stress Reduction:** Meditation is known for its ability to reduce stress by promoting relaxation and mindfulness. Chronic stress is linked to numerous health issues, including heart disease, high blood pressure, and weakened immune function. By reducing stress, meditation can help mitigate these risks, potentially leading to a longer life.

2. **Improved Cardiovascular Health:** Regular meditation practice has been associated with lower blood pressure and improved heart health. Studies suggest that meditation can enhance heart rate variability, a marker of cardiovascular health, and reduce the risk of heart disease.

3. **Enhanced Immune Function:** Meditation can boost the immune system by reducing stress hormones and increasing the production of antibodies. A stronger immune system can help protect against illnesses and infections, contributing to longevity.

4. **Better Mental Health:** Meditation has been shown to improve mental health by reducing symptoms of anxiety and depression. A positive mental state is crucial for overall well-being and can influence physical health, potentially extending lifespan.

5. **Cellular Aging:** Some studies suggest that meditation may have a positive impact on cellular aging. Telomeres, the protective caps on the ends of chromosomes, tend to shorten with age and stress. Meditation has been linked to increased telomerase activity, an enzyme that helps maintain telomere length, potentially slowing the aging process.

6. **Improved Sleep:** Quality sleep is essential for health and longevity. Meditation can improve sleep quality by promoting relaxation and reducing insomnia symptoms, leading to better overall health.

7. **Mind-Body Connection:** Meditation fosters a strong mind-body connection, encouraging individuals to be more attuned to their physical and emotional needs. This awareness can lead to healthier lifestyle choices, further supporting longevity.

Incorporating meditation into your daily routine can be a powerful tool for enhancing both mental and physical health, ultimately contributing to a longer and more fulfilling life.

Use your journal prompt and schedule into your diary some meditation time and feel the benefits. Head over to chapter 26 for more journal questions and take the time to embrace this fascinating powerful wellness tool.

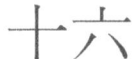

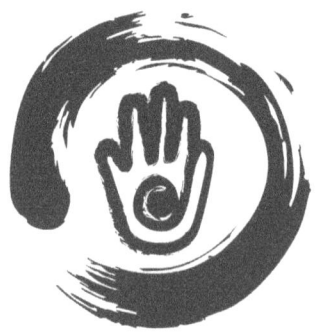

Dento Ryoho
Traditional Japanese Healing Practices
History, Science & Modern Adaptations

CHAPTER 16

Dento Ryoho - Traditional Japanese Healing Practices – History, Science & Modern Adaptations

During my years living in Japan, one of the most fascinating and enriching parts of daily life was witnessing how deeply healing is woven into Japanese culture. Wellness wasn't seen as a separate activity, it was part of how people cooked, moved, bathed, and connected. Healing was both preventative and restorative, drawing from centuries-old traditions that continue to influence modern practices today.

Let's explore the most respected and enduring traditional Japanese healing practices of Dento Ryoho 伝統療法, their historical roots, the growing body of science behind them, and how you can incorporate them into your own wellness journey.

1. **Kampo Medicine: Traditional Japanese Herbal Medicine**

History:

Kampo (漢方) originated from Traditional Chinese Medicine (TCM) and was adapted in Japan over 1,400 years ago. Unlike modern Western medicine that often isolates symptoms, Kampo treats the body holistically considering energy flow (Qi), blood circulation, and the balance of organ systems. Over time, Kampo evolved into its own uniquely Japanese form, with simplified formulas and a focus on symptom pattern recognition.

Science:

Today, Kampo is integrated into Japan's modern medical system and covered by national health insurance. Over 148 Kampo formulations are officially approved as prescription drugs in Japan. Research confirms the efficacy of certain Kampo herbs, such as *shosaiko-to* for liver support and *hochuekkito* for immune modulation and fatigue reduction.

Modern Adaptation:

You can explore Kampo-inspired herbal teas, adaptogenic tonics, or consult a practitioner trained in Japanese herbal therapy. It's also a reminder of how deeply healing can come from nature's pharmacy.

2. Shiatsu: The Art of Pressure Healing

History:

Shiatsu (指圧), meaning "finger pressure," is a therapeutic bodywork rooted in traditional Chinese acupressure but developed in Japan in the early 20th century. Practitioners use thumbs, palms, and elbows to apply rhythmic pressure along the body's meridians to release tension and stimulate energy flow (Qi or Ki).

Science:

Shiatsu has been shown in clinical studies to improve circulation, reduce cortisol levels, ease musculoskeletal pain, and enhance emotional well-being. One study published in the *Journal of Alternative and Complementary Medicine* found that regular shiatsu therapy significantly reduced symptoms of stress, fatigue, and back pain.

Modern Adaptation:

In Japan, shiatsu is often part of routine self-care. You can integrate its principles at home with self-massage, reflexology, or scheduling regular therapeutic sessions to support physical and emotional balance.

3. **Onsen (Hot Spring Therapy): Nature's Detox**

History:

Japan is a volcanic archipelago blessed with thousands of natural hot springs. For centuries, *onsen* bathing has been a cherished healing ritual for recovery, relaxation, and community bonding. Samurai would soak in hot springs to heal battle wounds, and temples often had access to sacred healing baths.

Science:

Onsen waters are rich in minerals like sulphur, magnesium, and calcium, known to relieve muscle and joint pain, improve skin conditions, and reduce inflammation. Immersion in hot water also increases circulation, aids in sleep, and supports parasympathetic nervous system activity, the body's "rest and digest" state.

Modern Adaptation:

You may not have access to a natural onsen but creating a bath ritual at home with magnesium flakes, Japanese hinoki oil (cypress), and mindful soaking can be a beautiful way to restore both body and spirit.

4. Reiki: Energy Healing with Global Reach

History:

Reiki (霊気) was developed by Mikao Usui in the early 20th century in Japan. The practice involves channelling life force energy (Ki) through the hands to promote healing, reduce stress, and balance the body's energy systems.

Science:

While Reiki is often considered a complementary therapy, emerging research shows promise. A 2019 systematic review in *Journal of Evidence-Based Integrative Medicine* found Reiki to be effective in reducing pain, anxiety, and depression in various populations. It's now practiced in hospitals, cancer centres, and wellness clinics worldwide.

Modern Adaptation:

You can explore Reiki through certified practitioners or even learn to self-practice. Many find it to be a meditative, spiritually grounding addition to daily wellness routines.

My Journey with Reiki: A Personal Experience

As a Reiki Master, my journey with energy healing has been profoundly transformative. Reiki, an ancient Japanese healing technique, has become an integral part of my life, offering a pathway to balance, peace, and well-being. It's like a little secret self-care ritual I do a few times a week to give myself a natural boost.

Personal Use and Self-Healing

My introduction to Reiki began with a desire to explore alternative healing methods for personal growth while living in Japan. Through regular practice, I discovered the profound impact Reiki had on my mental, emotional, and physical health. The gentle flow of energy during self-healing sessions brought a sense of calm and clarity, helping me navigate life's challenges with greater ease and resilience.

Reiki has become my go-to practice for maintaining balance in my daily life. Whether it's a quick session in the morning to set a positive tone for the day or a longer session in the evening to unwind, Reiki provides a sacred space for introspection and renewal. The practice has deepened my connection to my inner self, fostering a sense of empowerment and self-awareness.

A Lifelong Journey

My journey with Reiki is ongoing, continually evolving as I deepen my practice and understanding of energy healing. As a Reiki Master, I am committed to sharing this gift with others, empowering them to explore their own paths to healing and self-discovery.

Reiki has taught me that healing is not just about addressing physical ailments but embracing a holistic approach to well-being. It is a journey of self-discovery, connection, and transformation, one that I am grateful to share the world.

5. Forest Bathing (Shinrin-yoku): Immersion in Nature

History:

Originating in the 1980s in Japan as a public health initiative, *shinrin-yoku* or "forest bathing" encourages mindful immersion in nature not as exercise but simply being in the presence of trees and natural landscapes.

Science:

The Japanese government has funded years of research on the benefits of forest bathing. Studies from Tokyo's Nippon Medical School reveal that spending time in forests lowers blood pressure, reduces cortisol, and boosts immune function, particularly natural killer (NK) cells that fight cancer and infections.

Modern Adaptation:

Even if you don't live near forests, spending time in a garden, park, or by the sea while being mindful can provide similar effects. Add in breathwork and silence to amplify its healing power.

6. Moxibustion and Acupuncture: Traditional Energetic Therapies

History:

Both acupuncture and moxibustion (burning mugwort near or on specific points of the body) were adopted from China over

1,000 years ago and deeply ingrained into Japan's healing culture. Japanese acupuncture uses thinner needles and shallower insertion, making it gentler than the Chinese style.

Science:

Research shows acupuncture's effectiveness in treating chronic pain, anxiety, migraines, and hormonal imbalances. Moxibustion has been studied for boosting immune function and even correcting breech position in pregnancy.

Modern Adaptation:

If needles aren't your thing, try acupressure mats modern spins on ancient energetic practices.

A Holistic Philosophy of Healing

What makes Japanese healing practices unique is their integration of body, mind, spirit, and environment. They aren't isolated "treatments" but are connected to seasonal living, emotional regulation, and self-awareness. Healing isn't reactive—it's rhythmic and ritualistic.

By adopting even one or two of these traditions, you begin to tune your life to the rhythms of balance, harmony, and longevity.

Final note:

What traditional healing practice most intrigues you? Could you schedule a moment this week to explore or experience it?

Consider the role of belief in the healing process. How might being open to the possibility of healing, even if it's not something you currently subscribe to, affect your perspective or approach to challenges in life?

Write about any resistance or scepticism you might feel towards the idea of healing. What are the sources of these feelings, and how might exploring them lead to new insights or understandings?

Finally, reflect on how you can incorporate a sense of openness and curiosity about healing into your life. What small steps can you take to explore this concept further, whether through reading, conversations, or personal reflection?"

Use this prompt to delve into the concept of healing with an open mind, allowing yourself to explore new perspectives and possibilities, head over to the journal prompt in chapter 26 now.

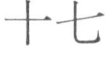

十七

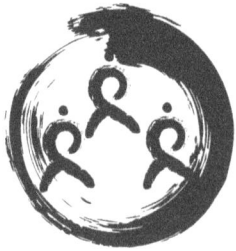

Kyōdōtai and Kizuna
The Power of Community and Connection in Japanese Culture

CHAPTER 17

Kyōdōtai and Kizuna — The Power of Community and Connection in Japanese Culture

In Japanese society, community and connection are not just conveniences they are cultural cornerstones. These values are expressed through beautifully nuanced language that reflects the importance of social harmony, mutual support, and emotional bonds. From ancient traditions to modern urban life, the Japanese understanding of human relationships can teach us how to cultivate stronger connections in our own lives.

Community in Japanese Culture

共同体 (Kyōdōtai) – *The Cooperative Body*

The word *kyōdōtai* reflects a traditional model of community where individuals work collectively toward a shared purpose. Rooted in agricultural and village life, this kind of community emphasizes mutual dependence and shared responsibility.

Everyone contributes, everyone belongs, and social cohesion is more important than individual ambition.

In a *kyōdōtai*, neighbours support one another through natural disasters, raise children together, and maintain public spaces with pride. Though modern life in Japan has shifted toward urban independence, the spirit of *kyōdōtai* is still deeply embedded in social expectations and civic life as seen in everything from school parent groups (*PTA*) to workplace harmony (*wa*).

地域社会 (Chiiki Shakai) – *The Local Society*

This term represents the more geographical side of community, like your town, neighbourhood, or region. *Chiiki shakai* still carries the implication of belonging, mutual care, and identity. Whether you live in a mountain village in Shikoku or a Tokyo high-rise, the Japanese tend to cultivate tight bonds with those in their immediate area. Local festivals (*matsuri*), volunteer clean-up days, and neighbourhood associations are not just activities, they are rituals of connection.

Connection and Emotional Bonds

絆 (Kizuna) – *The Invisible Thread*

Kizuna is a deeply emotional word, often translated as *bond* or *tie*. It evokes the invisible but unbreakable strings that hold people together, especially during difficult times. Following the 2011 Tōhoku earthquake and tsunami, *kizuna* became a national symbol of resilience. Families, strangers, and nations rallied together under this single, powerful word reminding everyone that connection is strength.

The sense of community that emerged in the aftermath of the Kobe earthquake, which was the most terrifying natural disaster I have ever personally experience, also known as the Great Hanshin Earthquake, on January 17th, 1995, was truly heartfelt and inspiring. In the wake of the 7.0 magnitude tremor, our neighbours immediately came together, offering vital support and resources. They provided us with water, food, and access to a telephone so we could reach out to our parents and loved ones.

Despite the overwhelming devastation, with nearly 90% of the community experiencing damage to their homes, there was an incredible spirit of unity and resilience. Everyone pitched in to help one another, demonstrating the strength and compassion that defined our community. This collective effort not only aided in our physical recovery but also reinforced the bonds between us, turning a time of crisis into a testament to human kindness and solidarity.

In everyday life, *kizuna* describes the warm ties between family, friends, coworkers, and even pets. It's the feeling of being held by something bigger than yourself. When you share a meal, offer help, or listen deeply, you nurture *kizuna*.

繋がり (Tsunagari) – *The Ongoing Link*

Tsunagari refers more broadly to the concept of being connected emotionally, socially, or even spiritually. It is the awareness that we are all linked, even across distances and differences. You'll often hear it used in wellness and mental health contexts to describe the importance of not feeling isolated.

With the rise of digital life, *tsunagari* has found new relevance in Japan. Even online communities strive to embody warmth and solidarity rather than anonymity. Whether through a neighbourhood group chat or a global community of ikebana enthusiasts, *tsunagari* helps people feel seen and supported.

Why This Matters to Wellness

Science confirms what these Japanese words express so poetically: strong social bonds and a sense of belonging are vital to our physical and mental health. Studies have shown that:

- Loneliness is as harmful to health as smoking 15 cigarettes a day.
- People with strong social connections live longer, experience less chronic disease, and have greater emotional resilience.
- Oxytocin, the "bonding hormone," is released during social interactions, helping regulate stress and improve heart health.

In Japanese culture, community and connection are preventative health tools—woven into the fabric of daily life. Whether it's joining a *moai* (a supportive friendship group in Okinawa), participating in tea ceremony, or simply saying *"otsukaresama deshita"* (thank you for your hard work) to colleagues, each gesture nurtures wellbeing.

How to Cultivate *Kyōdōtai, Kizuna,* and *Tsunagari* in Your Life

- Reach out regularly. Even a simple message can remind someone they're not alone.
- Join or create a group. Whether it's a book club, meditation circle, or walking group as shared purpose builds bonds.
- Give without expecting. A hallmark of Japanese social life is quiet generosity. Bake something. Offer help. Listen deeply.
- Celebrate rituals. Seasonal gatherings, shared meals, and birthdays offer natural moments to reconnect.

Japan teaches us that connection is not accidental, it is intentional, nurtured, and cherished. Whether it's the intimate bond of *kizuna*, the practical support of *kyōdōtai*, or the quiet web of *tsunagari* that links us across time and space, community is medicine. In a world that often glorifies independence, Japan reminds us that interdependence is where we truly thrive.

Now is the time to look at the journal prompts for this chapter and considered capturing your thoughts and experiences in a journal? It's a wonderful way to reflect on your journey not only in this chapter, but as you work your way through the book to explore your emotions and gain new insights. You might find it both relaxing and enlightening to put pen to paper and see where your thoughts take you. Why not give it a try and see what unfolds with the journal prompts for this chapter in chapter 26.

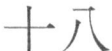

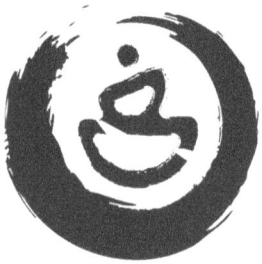

Kintsugi
Embracing Imperfection and Finding Beauty in the Broken

CHAPTER 18

Kintsugi - Embracing Imperfection and Finding Beauty in the Broken

Kintsugi 金継ぎ, meaning "golden joinery," is a profoundly beautiful and symbolic art form that transcends the boundaries of pottery and enters the realm of life philosophy. This Japanese practice involves repairing broken pottery, be it a cup, bowl, plate, or teapot with seams of gold, silver, or platinum. The result is not just a restored object, but a masterpiece that celebrates the imperfections, scars, and histories of the object. Rather than trying to hide the cracks, Kintsugi highlights them, transforming brokenness into a symbol of strength, resilience, and beauty.

The philosophy behind Kintsugi is rooted in the belief that breakage and imperfection are not to be viewed as flaws but as an inherent part of life's process. The idea is that when something breaks, it does not necessarily mean that it's the end. With the right care, attention, and time, it can be healed, not just restored, but transformed into something uniquely beautiful. This concept is a reflection of how Japanese culture views both physical and emotional damage, not as weaknesses, but as integral parts of one's journey that shape who we are.

In the process of Kintsugi, the cracks are filled with a lacquer mixed with powdered gold, which flows through the breaks, turning them into radiant, intricate patterns. The finished piece, now more beautiful and valuable than it was before its damage, becomes a symbol of resilience. The brokenness that was once seen as a flaw is now a feature to be admired. This is more than an art form, it is a profound lesson in how we, as humans, can heal our wounds, embrace our imperfections, and find strength in our scars.

I had the privilege of learning this beautiful art under the guidance of my pottery teacher, Mr. Tanaka, during my time living in Nara, Japan. I studied pottery with him for four years, and through this practice, I gained not only technical skills but also insights into the deeper philosophies that drive Japanese craftsmanship.

On one occasion, I brought in a broken tea bowl I had dropped during a rushed morning. As we worked through the painstaking process of restoration, my teacher said gently:

"This bowl now holds a story. It is stronger, more beautiful, and more valuable because it has been broken and mended."

Mr. Tanaka emphasized several life lessons through pottery and Kintsugi, lessons that resonate beyond the art of ceramics and can be applied to everyday life:

1. Admire Imperfection

In the Western world, we are often conditioned to believe that perfection is the ultimate goal, whether it's the flawless appearance of our homes, bodies, or careers. However, Japanese culture, and particularly Kintsugi, teaches us to appreciate imperfection. The cracks and imperfections in a pot are what give it character and uniqueness. It's the same with us: our flaws and scars are part of our story, and rather than hide them, we should honour them.

2. Always Do Your Best

This principle, called *shokunin kishitsu* (the spirit of craftsmanship), is deeply embedded in Japanese culture. It's the mindset of striving to do your best in everything, no matter how big or small the task may seem. In Kintsugi, the repair process requires patience, attention to detail, and a commitment to excellence, much like the way we should approach life, continuously seek improvement and striving for mastery in all we do.

3. Continuously Improve

The Japanese concept of *kaizen*, continuous improvement, is not only a practice for businesses but also a way of life. In the world of Kintsugi, as in life, there's always room for growth. Every pot that breaks and is repaired provides an opportunity to learn, adapt, and become better. The pursuit of improvement is constant, and the goal is not perfection but progress.

4. Make Your Talent a Gift to Others

Kintsugi is not about the artist's ego or fame. It's about the object being repaired and the joy it brings to others. In the same way, our talents and skills are meant to be shared, not hoarded. Whether it's through creating art, helping others, or offering our time and knowledge, we should aim to give back and contribute to the well-being of those around us. By sharing our gifts, we honour the interconnectedness of humanity and find deeper meaning in our work.

The practice of Kintsugi offers us a powerful metaphor for how to approach life. In a world that often feels focused on perfection and the avoidance of failure, Kintsugi reminds us that our cracks and scars, whether emotional, physical, or psychological, are not to be hidden. They are what make us who we are. Just as the gold in Kintsugi highlights the imperfections in pottery, our experiences, though sometimes painful, can be the very things that make us stronger, wiser, and more compassionate.

Incorporating Kintsugi into our lives doesn't mean simply mending broken pottery. It's about applying the principles of acceptance, patience, and appreciation of imperfection to our own experiences. When we experience setbacks, challenges, or heartbreak, we can choose to repair ourselves, honour our wounds, and emerge more beautiful and resilient than before.

Healing Through Imperfection: A Personal Journey

Reflecting on my time in Japan and my lessons with Mr. Tanaka, I've come to appreciate that the most significant growth often comes from moments of vulnerability and hardship. Just like the potter who repairs a broken piece of pottery, we, too, can heal our inner wounds with care and attention. We don't need to hide our scars or feel ashamed of them; instead, we can allow them to shine, to tell the story of our strength, and to teach us that beauty lies in the unique, the imperfect, and the real.

By embracing the art of Kintsugi, we can shift our perspective from seeking perfection to celebrating imperfection. We learn to value the beauty in life's cracks and to find strength in vulnerability. It's a philosophy that invites us to repair, rebuild, and restore, not just objects, but our very selves, transforming our brokenness into something radiant.

So, when life breaks us, as it inevitably does, we can choose to embrace our cracks, fill them with golden light, and emerge as something even more beautiful than before.

Kintsugi and Mental Well-Being

Kintsugi isn't just a poetic idea, it holds profound lessons for emotional healing and mental health.

1. Post-Traumatic Growth

Psychological studies have shown that people who experience hardship or trauma can experience post-traumatic growth—a concept very much aligned with Kintsugi. These individuals often develop greater inner strength, a deeper appreciation for life, and stronger relationships, much like a bowl reborn with golden seams.

2. Self-Compassion

Kintsugi encourages us to treat our own emotional wounds not with shame or denial, but with compassion and care. Just as the craftsman patiently restores each shard, we too can tend to our own healing process with gentleness.

3. Mindfulness and Ritual

The Kintsugi process requires time, precision, and attention. Every step,from collecting the broken pieces to applying the golden resin is meditative. Practicing Kintsugi or even reflecting on its philosophy can cultivate mindfulness, stillness, and the power of being present.

Kintsugi as a Wellness Practice

Even if you don't work with pottery, the metaphor of Kintsugi can be integrated into your daily life:

- Acknowledge your "cracks." Write about a challenging life event that left a mark on you. How did it change you?
- Celebrate your healing. What golden lessons came from this experience?
- Create a ritual. Whether it's journaling, creative expression, or even gentle stretching—practice something that honours your growth and resilience.

- Use art to process emotions. Many find that working with clay, gold paint, or collage can help externalize internal pain and start the journey of repair.

My Personal Kintsugi Journey

During my time in Japan, I had the privilege of learning Kintsugi from a master potter in Nara.

That lesson stayed with me. The process became a mirror for my own emotional healing, especially during life's turbulent chapters. Kintsugi helped me shift from self-criticism to self-honouring.

Final Note:

Kintsugi teaches us this: our scars are not shameful, they are sacred. In embracing them, we don't erase the past, we alchemize it. We become art.

So, the next time you feel broken, remember this:

'You are not damaged, you are becoming golden.'

Reflection Prompts

- In what areas of your life do you feel broken or imperfect? How might you begin to embrace and heal these parts of yourself, rather than hiding them?
- What are some of the "golden seams" in your life, the moments or experiences that have transformed you and made you stronger?

- How can you apply the principles of Kintsugi (admiring imperfection, continuous improvement, sharing your gifts) in your everyday life to cultivate greater resilience and beauty?

Take a moment to explore these journal prompts, designed to nurture your inner wellness and inspire meaningful actions. As you reflect, consider embracing the art of kintsugi by purchasing a kit online, complete with glue and gold leaf. This beautiful practice of repairing broken pottery, picture frames, or ornaments around your home symbolizes resilience and transformation, turning imperfections into unique works of art. Allow this creative process to mirror your journey of personal growth and healing.

Jump over to chapter 26 for more journal prompts for kintsugi.

十九

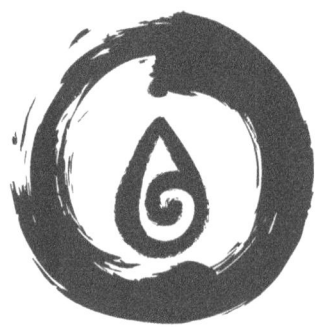

The Longevity Science of Ofuro
The Sacred Japanese Bathing Tradition

CHAPTER 19

The Longevity Science of Ofuro: The Sacred Japanese Bathing Tradition

I love having a bath, and I have so many fond memories and stories of bathing in Japan. In Japan, the ofuro (お風呂), a traditional Japanese bath, holds a deeply sacred place in daily life. It is more than just a routine, it's a ritual that embodies the perfect fusion of physical cleansing, mental relaxation, and spiritual renewal. While the act of bathing is common across cultures, the Japanese approach to bathing goes far beyond the mere need for cleanliness. It is a cultural practice that fosters longevity, promotes well-being, and helps maintain balance in life.

The ofuro involves soaking in a hot, deeply therapeutic bath, typically at temperatures ranging from 100°F to 110°F (38°C to 43°C), depending on individual tolerance. The bathing process is viewed as a form of self-care and mindfulness, where one's attention is given entirely to the experience of the bath and the sensation of warmth, the calming atmosphere, and the sound of water. This experience is not rushed but savoured, as Japanese tradition places a heavy emphasis on enjoying the present moment, making the ofuro a practice rooted in mindfulness and relaxation.

The Ritual of the Ofuro: More Than Just a Bath

Before stepping into the ofuro, it is customary to thoroughly cleanse the body. Bathers sit on small stools, using a hand-held showerhead or a gentle pouring bucket to wash away dirt and sweat. This ritual cleansing ensures that the bathwater remains pure and uncontaminated, which allows the soak itself to be deeply restorative.

The bath itself is a sacred time for reflection, solitude, and connection with one's body. In many Japanese households, the ofuro is located in a separate room from the rest of the house, creating a peaceful, quiet environment free of distractions. The water in the ofuro, often infused with natural scents such as yuzu or hinoki (Japanese cypress), creates an ambiance of relaxation, calming both the body and mind.

The Longevity Benefits of Ofuro

The tradition of ofuro bathing is more than just a luxurious indulgence—it is intertwined with scientific principles that support its role in promoting longevity and well-being. Several factors contribute to the profound benefits of the Japanese bath:

1. Stress Reduction and Mental Clarity

Soaking in warm water has been shown to reduce levels of cortisol, the hormone associated with stress. Chronic stress is a major contributor to a wide range of health issues, including heart disease, digestive problems, and weakened immunity. By providing a sanctuary of peace and relaxation, the ofuro bath offers a natural way to decompress from the pressures of daily life. The heat from the water promotes blood flow to the brain and encourages the production of endorphins—natural mood elevators. This helps to alleviate anxiety, calm the mind, and enhance overall mental well-being.

2. Improved Circulation

The heat from the bath causes blood vessels to dilate, which increases blood flow and enhances circulation. This improved circulation supports the body's ability to deliver oxygen and essential nutrients to the muscles and tissues, which in turn helps with the removal of toxins. Regular bathing in hot water has been shown to improve heart health by reducing blood pressure and supporting cardiovascular function. The relaxed state achieved through the ofuro can also reduce muscle tension and soreness, making it an excellent method for post-exercise recovery.

3. Detoxification and Skin Health

Soaking in hot water helps to open up the pores of the skin, allowing the body to release toxins and impurities. The act of sweating in the bath can aid in the detoxification process, promoting clearer, healthier skin. Many people in Japan find that regular ofuro bathing improves their complexion, as the warm water enhances the body's natural detoxifying processes. For those using aromatic oils or herbal infusions, such as yuzu, the water can also provide additional benefits by soothing the skin and reducing inflammation.

4. Enhanced Sleep Quality

The ofuro's relaxing effects can also improve sleep quality, which is a vital factor in maintaining good health and longevity. The calming effect of the warm water, combined with the meditative state fostered by the bathing process, can trigger the body's natural sleep cycle. After stepping out of the bath, the body temperature gradually lowers, signalling to the brain that it's time to rest. This drop in body temperature mimics the natural cooling process that occurs before sleep, promoting a deeper, more restful night's sleep.

5. Enhanced Immune Function

The soothing warmth of the ofuro stimulates the production of white blood cells, which play a critical role in the immune system. By encouraging circulation and promoting relaxation, regular bathing supports the body's ability to fight off infections and illnesses. In addition, the stress-reducing benefits of the bath help lower inflammation in the body, which is linked to chronic conditions like arthritis and autoimmune diseases.

6. **Emotional Healing and Mindfulness**

Bathing, particularly in the meditative atmosphere of the ofuro, offers profound emotional healing benefits. The uninterrupted time to focus solely on the sensation of the warm water enveloping the body creates space for introspection and emotional release. The practice of mindfulness, where the bather focuses on the present moment, can help to alleviate emotional strain and foster a deeper sense of connection with oneself. This mindful approach to bathing can enhance mental clarity, reduce negative thoughts, and contribute to a sense of emotional balance.

Scientific Studies on the Health Benefits of Hot Water Baths

Several scientific studies have investigated the benefits of hot water baths, many of which align with the principles of the ofuro tradition. For example, a study conducted by the Journal of Physiology and Pharmacology found that warm baths significantly improve blood circulation and cardiovascular health. Another study published in The European Journal of Applied Physiology demonstrated that soaking in hot water can improve muscle recovery and reduce inflammation, which is especially beneficial for those with chronic pain conditions or athletes.

In addition, research from Harvard Medical School has shown that regular hot baths can lower blood pressure, reduce the risk of heart disease, and even improve longevity. The practice of regular warm water baths is linked with better sleep quality, reduced stress levels, and improved mental health.

Incorporating Ofuro into Modern Life for Longevity

Incorporating the practice of ofuro-style bathing into our modern, fast-paced lives offers numerous benefits for physical and mental well-being. While many people may not have access to traditional Japanese hot springs (onsen), the concept of soaking in warm water and creating a calming ritual at home can be easily adapted. Consider setting aside time each evening to unwind in a warm bath, using calming scents like lavender or eucalyptus, and embracing the mindfulness aspect of the experience.

If you have access to an onsen or Spa, taking time to visit these places can provide not only the health benefits of the water but also the communal and restorative aspects of the practice. In Japan, the shared experience of bathing together in a public bath reinforces a sense of connection and community, contributing to the overall sense of well-being.

A Ritual of Longevity and Well-being

The tradition of the ofuro is far more than a daily habit; it is a ritual that has deep cultural, emotional, and health-related significance. The act of soaking in warm water is intertwined with mindfulness, relaxation, and a deep connection to the body and mind. The longevity science behind ofuro bathing demonstrates its profound effects on cardiovascular health, muscle recovery, stress reduction, and overall well-being.

By incorporating this sacred practice into modern life, we can foster a sense of calm, balance, and health that enhances our quality of life, supporting longevity and vitality as we age. Whether it's a quiet bath at home or a trip to an onsen, the practice of ofuro allows us to slow down, connect with ourselves, and heal—physically, mentally, and emotionally, one soak at a time.

Now is the perfect moment to dive into the journal prompts and carve out time for a rejuvenating bath, ofuro, or spa day with friends. Embrace the opportunity to unwind and experience the incredible benefits for yourself, nurturing both your body and spirit in the company of those you cherish.

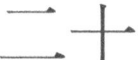

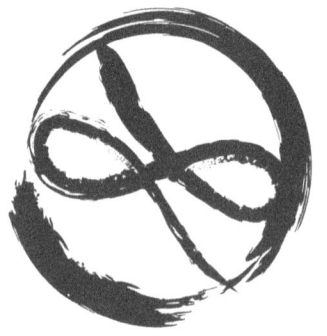

Shodo
The Way of Writing

CHAPTER 20

Shodo – The Way of Writing

Shodō (書道), which translates to *"the way of writing"*, is much more than beautiful handwriting—it is a profound, meditative art form rooted deeply in Japanese culture. This classical style of calligraphy dates back to ancient times, influenced by Chinese brush techniques and later evolving into a uniquely Japanese aesthetic that prizes not just precision, but presence, rhythm, and inner harmony.

In traditional Shodō, practitioners use a brush (*fude*), black ink (*sumi*), and rice paper (*washi*). The process begins with grinding an ink stick on a stone with water, a slow, mindful act that prepares both the materials and the mind. Then, with each brushstroke, the artist must be fully present. There's no room for correction, no second tries. Each mark reflects the artist's breath, energy, and state of mind in that moment.

Shodō is not about perfection. It's about expressing the spirit. The spaces between the strokes, the flow of the brush, and even the accidental splashes are embraced as part of the art.

This concept ties beautifully into the Japanese worldview of *wabi-sabi*, finding beauty in imperfection and transience.

The Science of Creative Flow

Modern neuroscience supports what Japanese culture has practiced for centuries. Engaging in focused creative practices like Shodō triggers a *flow state*, a mental zone where your brain becomes deeply immersed in the present. In this state, stress levels drop, the prefrontal cortex (responsible for overthinking and self-doubt) quiets, and feel-good neurotransmitters like dopamine and serotonin are released. This makes Shodō not just an artistic discipline, but a powerful tool for emotional regulation, mindfulness, and well-being.

Shodō in Everyday Life

You don't have to be a calligraphy master to enjoy the benefits. In my own life, I've adapted this tradition in simple and joyful ways. I find calm and creativity in Paint by Numbers, letting each colour and shape guide me into the same meditative space that brush and ink offer. But you can also:

- Write a handwritten letter of gratitude to someone you care about
- Try brush lettering or doodling a meaningful word or kanji character
- Make fun labels for the freezer or pantry
- Keep a daily ink journal with thoughts or sketches
- Try writing your *ikigai* or an intention for the day with slow, thoughtful strokes

The Spirit of Shodō

Ultimately, Shodō teaches us to slow down and connect with the brush, the paper, and ourselves. Each stroke is an invitation to pause and express something deeper than words. It's a reminder that the smallest daily rituals can become sacred, meaningful practices when approached with mindfulness.

So, whether you pick up a calligraphy brush or simply put pen to paper, let your writing become a meditative ritual. Find beauty in your lines, your loops, your scribbles and know that each one is an expression of your presence in the world.

Shodo calligraphy, the traditional Japanese art of writing, is deeply connected to the concept of longevity through its emphasis on mindfulness, discipline, and creativity. Here's how Shodo can contribute to a longer, more fulfilling life:

1. **Mindfulness and Focus**: Practicing Shodo requires a high level of concentration and presence, fostering a meditative state that can reduce stress and promote mental clarity. This mindfulness is beneficial for overall well-being and longevity.

2. **Stress Reduction**: Engaging in the rhythmic and deliberate movements of calligraphy can be calming and therapeutic, helping to lower stress levels, which is crucial for maintaining good health and extending one's lifespan.

3. **Discipline and Patience**: Shodo demands patience and discipline, qualities that are valuable in cultivating a balanced and resilient mindset. These traits can

enhance one's ability to navigate life's challenges, contributing to a longer, healthier life.

4. **Creativity and Expression**: The artistic nature of Shodo allows for personal expression and creativity, which can boost emotional well-being and provide a sense of fulfilment and purpose, key components of a long and satisfying life.

5. **Cultural Connection and Social Interaction**: Engaging in Shodo can also connect individuals to Japanese culture and history, fostering a sense of belonging and community. Participating in classes or groups can enhance social interactions, which are important for mental and emotional health.

By integrating Shodo into one's lifestyle, individuals can enjoy these holistic practises.

Journaling offers a unique opportunity to practice the art of Shodo, allowing you to connect deeply with the words you are writing. This practice invites you to slow down and let your thoughts flow naturally from your heart onto the paper. As you engage in this mindful activity, you are not only documenting your thoughts but also embracing the essence of Shodo, which emphasizes the beauty of each stroke and the intention behind every character.

By incorporating Shodo into your journaling routine, you create a space for reflection and self-expression. The deliberate and graceful movements of calligraphy encourage you to be present in the moment, fostering a sense of calm and clarity. This meditative process can help you gain insights into your emotions and experiences, promoting personal growth and understanding.

Moreover, the tactile experience of writing with a brush or pen enhances your connection to the words, making the act of journaling a more immersive and fulfilling practice. As you cultivate this connection, you may find that your journaling becomes a cherished ritual, offering both creative expression and a pathway to inner peace.

In essence, journaling through the lens of Shodo, transforms the simple act of writing into a profound journey of self-discovery and mindfulness, enriching your life with each thoughtful entry. Turn over to chapter 26 for more journal prompts about Shodo.

二十一

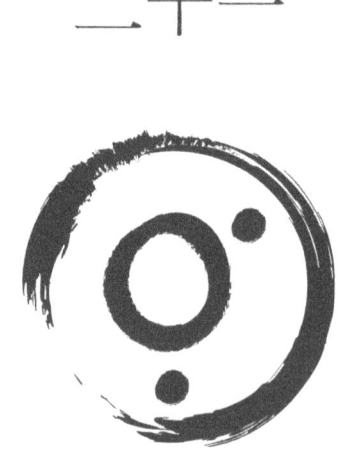

Ichigo Ichie
Once in a lifetime encounter

CHAPTER 21

Ichigo Ichie – Once in a lifetime encounter

Ichigo Ichie (一期一会) is a beautiful Japanese concept that translates to "one time, one meeting." It captures the fleeting nature of every moment and interaction, the idea that each encounter is unique and can never be replicated in quite the same way again. This mindset encourages presence, gratitude, and full attention to the here and now.

Origins and Philosophy

Ichigo Ichie finds its roots in the Japanese tea ceremony, where each gathering is treated as a once-in-a-lifetime event. The host meticulously prepares, and the guests enter with reverence, knowing that the same gathering will never occur again. Over time, this idea became a broader life philosophy appreciating every meal, conversation, sunrise, or smile as something to be cherished.

Ichigo Ichie and Wellness

Modern science now supports what Japanese tradition has always embraced: mindfulness and presence are crucial for mental and physical wellbeing.

- **Stress Reduction**: Focusing on the present reduces anxiety and rumination, key contributors to chronic stress and inflammation.
- **Emotional Health**: Gratitude and presence foster better emotional regulation and deeper relationships.
- **Longevity**: Studies show that mindfulness and social connection, core aspects of Ichigo Ichie are linked to improved immune function and longer life spans.

Daily Practice of Ichigo Ichie

- Start your day with awareness: greet the morning as a one-time gift. It is not guaranteed we get to see the following day, so be grateful for each morning we wake.
- When eating or drinking, focus entirely on taste, texture, and aroma. Have you ever noticed that each meal really is different, even if 2 different people are cooking from the same recipe.
- Listen to someone as if you'll never have this moment again. How would you listen differently, or how often do wish for another conversation with a loved one who has passed.
- Capture with your heart, not just your camera. Not every moment needs to be documented, put the phone

down, as some moments just need to be felt. Lock that feeling into your heart and mind!

This practice invites you to slow down, appreciate the ephemeral, and live with open-hearted awareness. By honouring each moment, we elevate daily life into a sacred ritual.

My first encounter with the phrase *Ichigo Ichie* came during one of my tea ceremony lessons in Japan. At the end of the session, my teacher gently guided me toward the *tokonoma*, the small alcove in her serene tearoom, where a piece of calligraphy hung, its brushstrokes elegant yet powerful. The characters read: 一期一会 (*Ichigo Ichie*).

She paused for a moment, letting the silence settle like steam over warm tea, and then softly explained its meaning: "This moment, this gathering, will never happen again in quite the same way. Even if we meet again, it will be different, because time moves, people change, and nothing repeats exactly."

That day, I truly felt the essence of *Ichigo Ichie*. It wasn't just a beautiful phrase; it was an invitation to be fully present. That tea ceremony, simple yet profound, became more than just a lesson in etiquette; it became a moment of stillness, connection, and awareness. I realized that this philosophy asks us to honour the uniqueness of every encounter, no matter how ordinary it may seem.

Since then, *Ichigo Ichie* has stayed with me as a quiet reminder to treat each moment as precious and unrepeatable, because it truly is.

Take a quiet moment to reflect on the precious encounters in your life, those once-in-a-lifetime moments that may never come again. What memories, feelings, or lessons surface as you think about *Ichigo Ichie*? Head over to the journal prompts in chapter 26 and honour the uniqueness of each experience by capturing it on the page.

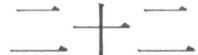

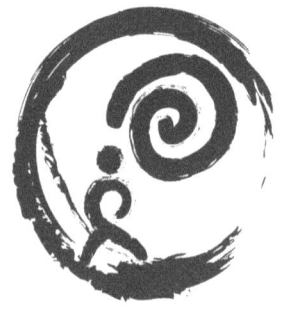

The Art of Japanese
Skincare & Wellness

CHAPTER 22

The Art of Japanese
Skincare & Wellness

In Japan, beauty isn't just skin-deep, it's deeply rooted in wellness, harmony, and ritual. The Japanese approach to skincare, スキンケア, is not about chasing perfection; it's about cultivating a peaceful relationship with your skin, your body, and your life. There are reasons Japanese women are renowned for their radiant, youthful complexions well into later life, this is the result of centuries-old traditions, mindful self-care, and a wellness philosophy that views beauty as a reflection of inner balance.

A Ritual, not a Routine

Skincare in Japan is treated as a slow, meditative ritual, often passed down through generations. Rather than hurriedly applying products, each step is performed with intention, creating a moment of calm and self-connection. Cleansing, for example, is not just about removing makeup, it's a time to massage the face, stimulate circulation, and release stress.

Applying lotion or essence becomes a nourishing act, rather than a chore.

This daily dedication contributes to many of the visible benefits of Japanese skincare rituals, including:

- Naturally lifted, toned facial muscles through massage-based cleansing techniques
- Fewer fine lines and wrinkles, as skin is kept hydrated, elastic, and gently stimulated
- Enhanced skin tone and radiance, supported by antioxidant-rich ingredients
- Reduced puffiness and stress-related facial tension, especially around the jaw, brow, and under-eyes
- Greater self-awareness and mindfulness, promoted through slow, mindful movements

The Science Behind the Glow

Several modern studies support the effectiveness of Japanese beauty practices for both wellness and dermatological health:

Facial Massage & Lymphatic Drainage

One of the key techniques in Japanese skincare is facial massage, often incorporated during cleansing or moisturizing. This helps increase blood flow, improve lymphatic drainage, and reduce puffiness. A 2018 study published in *PLoS One* showed that regular facial massage increased skin elasticity and improved facial contour over a 4-week period.

Massage also stimulates the parasympathetic nervous system, helping reduce cortisol levels (the stress hormone) and creating a sense of calm.

Ingredients Rooted in Nature

Japanese skincare heavily features natural, antioxidant-rich ingredients, many of which have stood the test of time and are now backed by science:

- **Green tea (matcha)** – Packed with catechins, green tea reduces inflammation and neutralizes free radicals. A 2013 study in *Journal of the American Academy of Dermatology* noted that green tea extract improves acne and reduces sun damage.
- **Rice bran** – Rich in ferulic acid and squalene, it helps protect the skin barrier and maintain moisture.
- **Seaweed (kombu, wakame)** – Loaded with minerals and polysaccharides that hydrate and protect the skin from environmental damage.
- **Camellia oil (tsubaki)** – High in oleic acid and vitamin E, this traditional moisturizer deeply nourishes and improves skin elasticity.
- **Mindfulness & Cortisol Reduction**

Mindful rituals like skincare, bath time (*ofuro*), and facial yoga activate the rest-and-digest system, promoting cellular repair and reducing systemic inflammation. Lower cortisol levels are directly linked to slower skin aging, better sleep, and improved immune response.

Modern Adaptations with Ancient Roots

Today, you'll find a growing global interest in Japanese skincare principles, from *double cleansing* to *essence layering* and *gua sha-style massage*. Yet the essence remains unchanged: slowness, purity, and presence. Rather than overloading the skin with harsh products, Japanese rituals focus on strengthening and supporting the skin's natural function.

A Wellness Practice in Disguise

Many people approach skincare as a form of vanity. But in the Japanese philosophy, it's about nourishment, harmony, and respect, not just for your face, but for your whole being. You are not just applying a cream; you're grounding yourself, observing your own needs, and caring for yourself in a deeply intentional way.

When you engage in this kind of practice daily, the effects ripple outward, not just in glowing skin, but in how you feel in your body, how you handle stress, and how you show up in the world.

Japanese beauty rituals are deeply rooted in tradition, nature, and minimalism, and many of them focus on prevention, balance, and consistency rather than quick fixes. Here are some of the most respected and effective Japanese beauty rituals that contribute to youthful, glowing skin:

1. **Double Cleansing**

   - **Ritual**: Start with an oil-based cleanser to remove makeup, sunscreen, and impurities, followed by a gentle foaming cleanser to clean deeper into the pores.
   - **Why it works**: Prevents clogged pores and ensures your skin is truly clean without stripping it.
   - **Cultural roots**: This method is inspired by the geisha tradition, who used natural oils to remove heavy makeup before cleansing with rice water.

2. **Green Tea (Matcha) Beauty**

   - **Ritual**: Drinking green tea daily and using green tea–infused skincare.
   - **Why it works**: Green tea is rich in antioxidants (especially EGCG), which help reduce inflammation, fight free radicals, and slow aging.
   - **How to try**: Use matcha face masks, toners, or serums, and drink fresh-brewed green tea.

3. **Rice Water Rinse**

   - **Ritual**: Using the water leftover from rinsing rice to wash the face or as a toner.
   - **Why it works**: Rice water is packed with vitamins, amino acids, and minerals that soften, brighten, and nourish the skin.
   - **Science**: Rice bran is rich in ferulic acid and allantoin, known for anti-aging and soothing benefits.

4. **Layering Lightweight Hydration**

- **Ritual**: Applying hydrating layers (lotions, essences, and serums) from thinnest to thickest, rather than using one heavy cream.
- **Why it works**: Keeps skin plump, dewy ("mochi skin"), and allows each product to absorb better without clogging pores.

5. **Daily Facial Massage**

- **Ritual**: Gently massaging the face with the fingers or a tool (like a gua sha or kansa wand).
- **Why it works**: Boosts circulation, reduces puffiness, promotes lymphatic drainage, and helps prevent sagging.

6. **Less is More Philosophy**

- **Ritual**: Using only a few high-quality products rather than overwhelming the skin.
- **Why it works**: Reduces the risk of irritation and keeps the skin's barrier healthy.
- **Japanese phrase**: *"Hadanashi"* – a minimalist approach to skincare.

7. **Regular Onsen and Ofuro Soaking**

- **Ritual**: Bathing in mineral-rich hot springs or at home in a deep, relaxing bath.

- **Why it works**: The minerals (like sulphur and magnesium) detoxify the skin, while the heat increases blood flow and helps with cell renewal.

8. **Nighttime Skincare Rituals**

   - **Ritual**: Emphasis on evening routines with focus on cleansing, hydration, and relaxation.
   - **Why it works**: Skin regenerates during sleep, so preparing it well before bed is key.
   - **Extra tip**: Many Japanese women sleep on silk pillowcases to reduce friction and wrinkles.

9. **Sun Protection is Sacred**

   - **Ritual**: Wearing SPF daily, rain or shine. Hats, umbrellas, and UV-protective clothing are also common.
   - **Why it works**: Prevents sun damage, which is the number 1 cause of premature aging.

10. **Japanese Facial Yoga**

Often called "face yoga" or "facial exercises" is a natural beauty practice rooted in traditional Japanese self-care, designed to tone, lift, and rejuvenate the facial muscles through specific movements and expressions. It combines gentle massage, stretching, acupressure, and breathing techniques to stimulate circulation, release tension, and promote youthful, glowing skin.

Key Concepts of Japanese Facial Yoga

1. Activate Underused Facial Muscles
   o The face has over 40 muscles, many of which we don't actively use.
   o Facial yoga tones and strengthens these muscles to prevent sagging and promote definition especially around the jawline, cheeks, and eyes.
2. Boost Circulation & Lymphatic Flow
   o Gentle massage and tapping help oxygenate the skin and reduce puffiness.
   o This detoxifying effect gives the skin a healthy glow and can help diminish dark circles and dullness.
3. Relieve Tension
   o We carry stress in our face (clenching jaws, furrowing brows).
   o Facial yoga promotes relaxation, softens expression lines, and reduces the signs of emotional stress.
4. Stimulate Collagen Production
   o Through regular movement and pressure, the skin is encouraged to produce more collagen and elastin, vital for youthful firmness and elasticity.

Common Japanese Facial Yoga Techniques

- "O" and "Smile" Movements: Tone cheeks and jawline
- Eye Lifting: Gently pressing above the brow and lifting eyes upward
- Neck & Jaw Stretching: Prevents sagging and double chin

- Facial Tapping & Lymph Drainage Massage: Boosts circulation and detox

Wellness & Skincare Benefits

- Naturally lifted, toned face
- Fewer fine lines and wrinkles
- Enhanced skin tone and radiance
- Reduced puffiness and stress-related tension
- Greater self-awareness and mindfulness

Incorporating It into Your Ritual

Skincare Meets Self-Care: Try This Mini Ritual

1. **Cleanse slowly**, massaging the skin with circular motions.
2. **Apply a toner or essence** with your palms, pat it gently into your skin, focusing on how it feels.
3. **Use a jade roller or fingertips** to massage a facial oil into your skin, paying attention to the tension points (jawline, temples, under the eyes).
4. **Breathe deeply** throughout, anchoring yourself in the present.
5. **Smile at yourself** in the mirror when you're done— your presence is your beauty.

You only need 5–10 minutes a day to begin seeing results. Combine it with your skincare routine right after cleansing or while applying oil or serum for a deeply relaxing and restorative ritual.

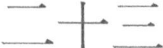

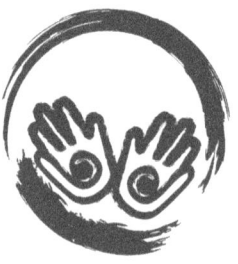

Integrating Japanese Wellness
Wisdom into Modern Life for Longevity

CHAPTER 23

Integrating Japanese Wellness Wisdom into Modern Life for Longevity

Living a long, vibrant, and fulfilling life doesn't require drastic change, it requires intentional living, small consistent habits, and a grounded connection to the people and world around you. Japan, particularly regions like Okinawa (a renowned Blue Zone), offers a holistic blueprint for longevity rooted in ancient practices, cultural values, and daily rituals.

Across this book, we've explored Japanese wellness through the lens of food, movement, minimalism, mindfulness, nature, community, and emotional connection. Now, it's time to bring it all together and make it part of your own life—one that prioritizes health, calm, and joy.

The Pillars of Japanese Wellness at a Glance

1. Wabi-Sabi & Kanso – Embrace simplicity, imperfection, and mindful living. Let go of clutter (mental and physical) to create space for peace.
2. Nutrition & The Okinawan Diet – Focus on seasonal, plant-forward eating, moderate portions (*hara hachi bu*), and nourishing your body with variety and intention.
3. Movement – Integrate joyful, sustainable movement like walking, gentle stretching, and traditional arts like *tai chi* or *radio taisō*.
4. Mindfulness & Meditation – Prioritize stillness with Zen meditation (*zazen*), forest bathing (*shinrin-yoku*), or tea ceremonies for daily presence.
5. Ikigai – Discover your purpose. Even small passions can give you the motivation to rise each day with meaning.
6. Community & Connection – Strengthen your *kizuna* (bonds), lean into support, and build community around shared values (*kyōdōtai*).
7. Creativity & Ritual – From *ikebana* to calligraphy and tea preparation, engage in rituals that slow time and reconnect you with beauty.
8. Traditional Healing & Prevention – Integrate natural remedies, massage, food therapy, and preventive health as part of self-care.

Bringing the Wisdom into Your Daily Life

Here are some ways to gently incorporate Japanese wellness into a modern, often fast-paced life:

1. Start Small & Build Rituals

Rather than overhaul your lifestyle, choose one habit that resonates. Perhaps it's drinking green tea mindfully each morning, walking slowly through nature, or adding one more vegetable to your plate.

2. Design Your Space with Purpose

Let *kanso* guide your home's energy. Clear your space of what no longer serves you. A clean and intentional space supports a clear mind.

3. Live with Awareness

Practice *zazen* or simply sit for 5 minutes a day in silence. Let your breath be your anchor. Over time, this cultivates calm, presence, and emotional resilience.

4. Nourish Your Body Like It Matters

Follow the Okinawan principle: Eat more plants, less sugar, and stop at 80% full. Cook more often, slow down, and eat with appreciation.

5. Connect on Purpose

Whether through family dinners, community groups, or heartfelt messages, invest time in people who uplift and energize you. Strong emotional bonds increase longevity and protect against disease.

6. Create & Contribute

Channel your *ikigai*—something you love, are good at, and can offer the world. It doesn't have to be big. Even tending a garden, journaling, or volunteering once a week gives life meaning.

7. Honour the Seasons

Align your habits with nature. Seasonal eating, seasonal cleaning, and seasonal reflection keep you grounded and adaptable.

The Science Behind Longevity

Modern science supports what traditional Japanese culture has long known:

- Community reduces stress and lowers the risk of heart disease, stroke, and dementia.
- Plant-based diets lower inflammation, improve metabolic health, and prevent chronic illness.
- Mindfulness and meditation rewire the brain, reduce anxiety, and increase focus and compassion.
- Purpose (ikigai) is associated with lower mortality rates and improved quality of life.
- Gentle movement improves joint health, mood, and cognition, especially in aging populations.

A Life of Gentle Balance

You don't have to live in a small Japanese village or attend daily tea ceremonies to benefit from these ancient teachings. The essence of Japanese wellness is about living slowly, intentionally, and connected to what matters most, your health, your people, your values, and your environment.

My weekly routine (take inspiration and start your own routine)

This personal daily regime that incorporates these rich Japanese concepts and practices can be a transformative experience. Here's a suggested schedule for one week, designed to nurture your mind, body, and spirit: For the meals, choose from the 15 recipes, or be creative and experiment with healthy Japanese ingredients yourself.

Day 1: Mindful Beginnings

- **Morning**: Start with a meditation session focused on wabi-sabi, appreciating the beauty in imperfection and transience.
- **Breakfast**: Enjoy a traditional Japanese breakfast with miso soup, grilled fish, and rice.
- **Mid-Morning**: Practice Shodo calligraphy, focusing on a word that resonates with your current state of mind. This is perfect for breaktime (Shodo notebook, and pen in my handbag for a 15-minute break to clear my head and concentrate on something to support my mental health)
- **Lunch**: a nourishing lunch

- **Afternoon**: Engage in a green tea ceremony, savouring each step and moment.
- **Dinner**: meal plan a nourishing dinner
- **Evening**: Reflect on your day with journaling, incorporating thoughts on gaman (endurance) and resilience.

Day 2: Creative Exploration

- **Morning**: Begin with a light exercise routine, such as yoga or tai chi, to energize your body.
- **Breakfast**: Prepare a healthy smoothie with matcha and seasonal fruits.
- **Mid-Morning**: Create an ikebana arrangement, focusing on simplicity and harmony.
- **Lunch**: a healthy lunch inspired by Japanese ingredients
- **Afternoon**: Explore your ikigai by writing about what brings you joy and purpose.
- **Dinner**: meal plan healthy dinners
- **Evening**: Practice/Learn/have a treatment from a Reiki practitioner on yourself, focusing on healing and balance.

Day 3: Continuous Improvement

- **Morning**: Meditate on the concept of kaizen, setting small goals for personal growth.
- **Breakfast**: Enjoy a bowl of oatmeal topped with nuts and fruits.
- **Mid-Morning**: Engage in a kintsugi project, repairing a broken item with gold leaf.

- **Lunch**: a healthy Japanese inspired lunch
- **Afternoon**: Take a mindful walk, appreciating the present moment (Ichigo Ichie).
- **Dinner**: healthy planned dinner
- **Evening**: Indulge in a beauty ritual, such as a facial mask or bath, to relax and rejuvenate.

Day 4: Balance and Harmony

- **Morning**: Start with a meditation session focusing on balance and harmony.
- **Breakfast**: Have a simple meal of steamed vegetables and rice.
- **Mid-Morning**: Practice Shodo, writing characters that symbolize balance.
- **Lunch**: a healthy Japanese inspired lunch
- **Afternoon**: Participate in a green tea ceremony, inviting a friend to share the experience.
- **Dinner**: plan for healthy dinners
- **Evening**: Reflect on your day with journaling, focusing on moments of harmony and balance.

Day 5: Inner Strength

- **Morning**: Begin with a strength-training exercise routine.
- **Breakfast**: Prepare a protein-rich meal with tofu and vegetables.
- **Mid-Morning**: Engage in an ikebana session, using flowers that symbolize strength and resilience.
- **Lunch**: experiment with healthy Japanese ingredients

- **Afternoon**: Explore your ikigai by identifying activities that align with your values.
- **Evening**: Practice Reiki, focusing on areas where you seek strength and healing and have an ofuro before bed as part of your bedtime routine

Day 6: Mindful Reflection

- **Morning**: Meditate on the concept of Ichigo Ichie, appreciating each unique moment.
- **Breakfast**: Enjoy a traditional Japanese breakfast with vegetables, tofu or salmon and rice.
- **Mid-Morning**: Work on a kintsugi project, reflecting on the beauty of repaired items.
- **Lunch**: keep eating a variety of healthy Japanese style ingredients
- **Afternoon**: Take a mindful walk, observing the beauty in your surroundings.
- **Dinner**: make a new inspiring recipe
- **Evening**: Indulge in a beauty ritual, such as a soothing bath with essential oils.

Day 7: Integration and Celebration

- **Morning**: Start with a meditation session, integrating all the week's practices.
- **Breakfast**: Have a celebratory meal with your favourite healthy Japanese dishes.
- **Mid-Morning**: Reflect on your journey through journaling, focusing on personal growth and insights.
- **Lunch**: be creative with healthy ingredients

- **Afternoon**: Host a green tea ceremony with friends, celebrating the week's experiences.
- **Dinner**: meal plan with healthy ingredients and eat something different each day.
- **Evening**: Conclude with a Reiki session, focusing on gratitude and peace, then before bed, have an ofuro to set you up for a great sleep.

This schedule is designed to be flexible, allowing you to adapt each day's activities to your personal preferences and needs. Enjoy the journey of integrating these enriching practices into your daily life!

二十四

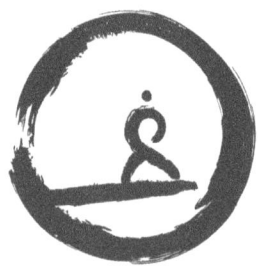

Japanese
Inspired Travel Routine
for Wellness & Longevity

CHAPTER 24

Japanese-Inspired Travel Routine for Wellness & Longevity

Before You Travel – Grounding Preparation

1. **Pack with Rituals in Mind**

   - **Miniatures of comforts**: Pack travel-size skincare (rice water toner, green tea mist), facial massage tools, a silk eye mask, and essential oils (like yuzu or hinoki).
   - **Tea sachets**: Bring green tea or hojicha for calming digestion and staying grounded.
   - **Journal**: Carry a small notebook for Ichigo Ichie reflections, gratitude, or Shodo-inspired sketching.
   - **Healthy snacks**: Edamame packs, seaweed snacks, miso sachets, or onigiri if possible.

2. **Pre-flight Ofuro-Inspired Shower or Bath**

   - Before heading to the airport, have a long warm soak or steamy shower with Japanese bath salts or hinoki-scented body wash. This relaxes the nervous system and sets a calming tone.

In Transit – Calm in Chaos

1. **Mindful Movement – "Kansha Tai Sō" (Gratitude Exercise)**

   - Gentle stretches or Seiza (kneeling meditation) before boarding, actually I do this just seated by the boarding gate so I just look like I'm having a stretch and closing my eyes resting, little does anyone know….
   - On the plane/train: Ankle rolls, neck rolls, hand stretches, or brief standing stretches every 2 hours.

2. **Facial Yoga & Lymphatic Massage (Japanese Beauty Practice)**

   - Use fingers or a gua sha tool to relieve puffiness, improve circulation, and refresh your face mid-flight.

3. **Japanese-Inspired Nourishment (Eiyōshoku)**

   - Skip the heavy plane food when possible. Choose simple, whole foods:
     - Miso soup if available
     - Green tea
     - Rice + veggies + protein combo
     - Avoid sugary drinks and processed snacks

4. **Sensory Anchors – Ichigo Ichie on the Move**

- Pause during transit moments (boarding, looking out the window, a kind interaction). Remind yourself: *"This moment is once-in-a-lifetime."*
- Jot down quick reflections: *What feels beautiful right now? What am I grateful for?*

At Your Destination – Restore Balance

1. **Quick Hotel Room Ritual – Create a Zen Space**

- Open a window if you can and breathe deeply.
- Set up a mini ritual corner with tea, mist, your journal, or a photo.
- Light stretching or Tai Chi-inspired flow for 5–10 minutes.

2. **Kanso & Decluttering Mindset**

- Keep your travel space tidy. Unpack a little. Store excess. Calm environment = calm mind.

3. **Bathing Ritual (Mini Ofuro)**

- Hot shower in the evening with intentional slowness. Add bath salts if available.
- Use a washcloth to exfoliate—Japanese-style—while being mindful of breath and movement.

4. **Skin & Sleep Care (Beauty + Longevity)**

- Double cleanse (if you can), apply rice water toner or green tea mist, and moisturize.
- Use facial massage to release tension.
- Sleep early, if possible, rest is a foundation of Japanese wellness.

Eating While Traveling – Shojin Ryori-Inspired Mindfulness

1. **Choose Balanced Plates When Eating Out**

- Prioritize: vegetables, rice, miso, seaweed, and fish if possible.
- Practice *Hara Hachi Bu*: eat until you're 80% full.

2. **Enjoy Without Guilt—Ichigo Ichie at Mealtimes**

- If you do have a buffet or indulgence, enjoy it slowly and fully. Every meal is a moment. Be present.

Closing Each Day – Reflection & Calm

1. **Gratitude & Kintsugi Metaphor**

- Write about a challenge or travel mishap and how it added to the richness of the experience.
- Ask yourself: *Where did I find beauty in imperfection today?*

2. Short Meditation or Breathing Practice (Zazen-style)

- Sit still for just 3–5 minutes. Focus on your breath. Be here now.

Travel will always present disruptions but with a few adaptable Japanese rituals, you can transform your time away into a meaningful, mindful experience that nourishes your body, skin, and spirit.

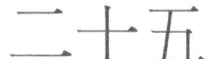

二十五

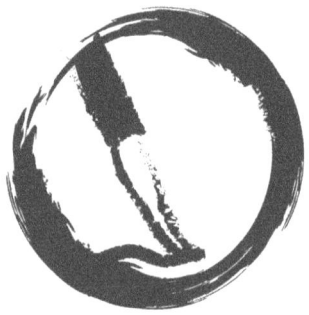

Final note from Barbara

CHAPTER 25

Final note from Barbara

A Gentle Invitation to Live Well, Every Day

Let this final chapter be not just an ending, but a beginning, your invitation to weave ancient Japanese wisdom into the fabric of your everyday life. My journey began over a decade ago in Japan, where I was deeply moved by the elegance and intentionality of daily living. What I discovered there changed me. And now, through these pages, I've shared that journey with you.

You don't need to master every ritual or follow every tradition. Begin where you are. Choose what resonates with your heart. Maybe it's preparing a nourishing bowl of miso soup, lighting incense before journaling, or simply pausing to appreciate the fleeting beauty of a sunrise. Over time, these small, deliberate acts of self-respect and presence build a life that is not only longer, but richer, deeper, and more meaningful.

In a world that moves quickly and often demands more than we can give, the quiet, timeless rituals of Japan offer us a way home, to ourselves, to nature, and to what truly matters. These practices are not just about health or beauty or even longevity. They are about connection. Presence. Grace. A sense of reverence for the ordinary.

Whether it's:

- the meditative breath of *zazen*,
- the healing warmth of an *ofuro* bath,
- the mindful bite of a simple *shōjin ryōri* meal,
- the emotional depth of *kintsugi* restoration, or
- the soulful clarity found in a calligraphy stroke of *shodō*—

Each ritual whispers the same gentle message:

Slow down. Be here. You are enough.

Wellness, the Japanese way, is not a performance, it is a practice. It is not found in extremes, but in quiet, daily devotion to simplicity, nourishment, movement, connection, and self-awareness. It reminds us that true vitality comes from harmony within ourselves, with others, and with the world around us.

You don't need to live in Japan to live with Japanese wisdom.

All it takes is intention. And kindness.

Start small. Pick one ritual that speaks to your soul. Maybe it's writing a letter of gratitude. Maybe it's choosing *hara hachi bu* at your next meal try eating to 80% fullness. Maybe it's taking five minutes of stillness in the morning before the noise of the day begins. Let that ritual anchor you. Let it reconnect you.

From there, these practices will begin to grow roots, transforming your routine into a rhythm, your space into a sanctuary, and your life into a reflection of care.

And when you look back, you'll find that the journey to wellness and longevity wasn't a sprint.

It was a walk. A slow, steady, beautiful walk, blossoming like *sakura* in spring.

Thank you for walking it with me.

Arigatō gozaimashita.
With love,
Barbara Lovesy

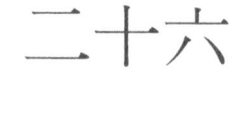

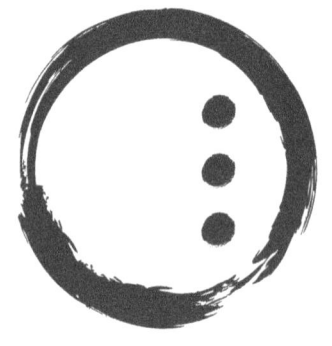

Journal Prompts

CHAPTER 26

Journal Prompts

Welcome to your personal sanctuary, a space to slow down, reflect, and reconnect with yourself.

This journal part of the book is inspired by the time-honoured traditions of Japanese wellness, where simplicity, nature, and mindfulness are woven into everyday life. From the calming practice of *shodo* (calligraphy) to the nourishing rituals of *ofuro* (bathing), and the soulful art of *kintsugi* (golden repair), each chapter you've explored offers more than a practice—it offers a philosophy of living with intention and grace.

Here, you are invited to pause, breathe deeply, and write. Let these pages be where your thoughts unfold, your insights deepen, and your personal journey towards balance and longevity is lovingly recorded.

Whether you are sipping green tea, arranging flowers, or simply sitting in stillness, may your reflections guide you to a deeper sense of wellness—one that is grounded in self-respect, connection, and joy.

Let this journal be your companion as you integrate these beautiful Japanese traditions into your modern life, one mindful moment at a time.

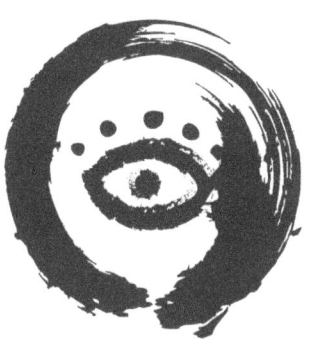

Wabi–Sabi
Admire Imperfection

Journal Prompts: for Chapter 1.
Wabi-Sabi – Admire Imperfection

Reset Your Way of Thinking

- What is one belief or expectation I can let go of today?
- Where in my life am I holding on to perfectionism?
- What does imperfection mean to me and how can I begin to see beauty in it?

Trade Judgement for Acceptance

- When was the last time I judged myself harshly? What would it feel like to replace that judgement with compassion?
- What parts of myself do I find hardest to accept? Why?

- How would my life shift if I focused more on *progress* than *perfection*?

Forgive

- Who do I need to forgive either someone else or myself?
- What has holding onto resentment cost me emotionally or physically?
- What would forgiveness free me to do or feel?

Stop Comparing

- Who do I often compare myself to, and what does that reveal about my own insecurities?
- What do I have right now that someone else might be wishing for?
- How can I celebrate my own unique journey today?

Simplify

- What areas of my life feel cluttered physically, emotionally, or mentally?
- What is one small thing I can remove or reduce to create space for peace?
- Where in my routine can I add more calm and less chaos?

Work on Self-Acceptance

- Write a letter to your younger self highlighting what you love and admire about them now.

- What are 3 things I genuinely appreciate about myself today?
- If I treated myself like someone I love, how would I speak, act, and think differently?

Look at Wisdom as Beauty

- What experience in my life, though painful, has made me wiser?
- How has age or time shaped me in beautiful ways?
- What does "beauty through growth" mean to me?

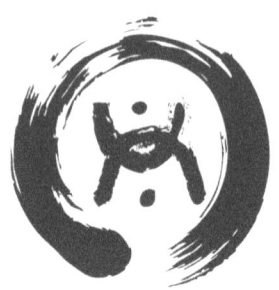

Gaman
Live with Great Resilience

Journal Prompts: Chapter 2. Gaman – Live with Great Resilience

Take Action

- What is one small action I've been avoiding, and how can I take the first step today?
- What does "taking action" look like when I'm afraid or uncertain?
- When have I felt empowered by taking initiative, no matter how small?

Eat Fresh

- How does eating fresh, whole foods affect my energy and mood?
- What's one healthy food I enjoy that I can eat more often?

- How can I make preparing meals a more mindful and nourishing experience?

Cut Back

- Where in my life can I practice restraint or moderation?
- What do I consume too much of (e.g., social media, sugar, news), and how does it impact my wellbeing?
- What's one area I can simplify this week for greater peace of mind?

Get Moving

- What physical activity makes me feel most alive and connected to my body?
- How can I bring more joyful movement into my daily routine?
- When I move my body, what emotions do I notice?

Socialize in Real Life

- Who do I feel truly seen and supported by in my life?
- How does in-person connection affect my emotional health?
- What's one meaningful connection I can nurture more intentionally?

Work Out

- What motivates me to stay physically strong and resilient?

- How does working out help me handle stress or adversity?
- How do I define strength—both physically and emotionally?

Meditate

- What comes up for me when I sit in stillness?
- How does meditation help me respond (instead of react) to stress?
- What would 5 minutes of mindful breathing do for me right now?

Make Peace

- What or whom do I need to make peace with?
- How does holding on to conflict or regret weigh me down?
- What does peace feel like in my body, and how can I return to it more often?

Stay the Course

- What goal or value is worth staying the course for, even when it's hard?
- How have I shown resilience in the past, and what did I learn from it?
- What daily habits keep me grounded and focused on my long-term wellbeing?

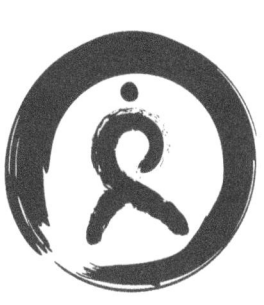

Eiyoshoku
Nourish Your Body

Journal Prompts: Chapter 3. Nourishing Your Body with Eiyōshoku

1. **How does the food I eat make me feel—physically, mentally, and emotionally?**
   (Reflect on the connection between your meals and your energy, mood, or focus.)

2. **What does "nourishment" mean to me beyond calories or nutrients?**
   (Is it about warmth, preparation, intention, or the memory attached to a dish?)

3. **Which Japanese eating habits could I adopt to feel more energized or balanced?**
   (Consider mindful eating, smaller portions, more variety, or seasonal foods.)

4. **What are 3 ingredients I could include more often to support my health? Why?**

(Think of antioxidant-rich foods like seaweed, green tea, miso, tofu, or mushrooms.)

5. **When was the last time I slowed down and truly appreciated a meal?**

   (Write about what made it special—who you were with, what you ate, how you felt.)

6. **How can I bring more intention into my meals this week?**

   (Examples: cooking at home, expressing gratitude before eating, eating without screens.)

7. **What food rituals from my childhood or culture bring me a sense of comfort or care?**

   (Explore how to reintroduce or modernize them in your current life.)

8. **What limiting beliefs do I hold around food and nourishment? How can I shift them?**

   (For example: "I don't have time to cook" or "Healthy food isn't satisfying.")

9. **In what ways can I use food as an act of self-love rather than control or punishment?**

   (Reflect on how to move toward a more gentle and respectful relationship with your body.)

10. **Write a food mantra or affirmation to guide your approach to nourishing your body.**

    (E.g., "I choose foods that make me feel alive." or "My meals are a gift to my body.")

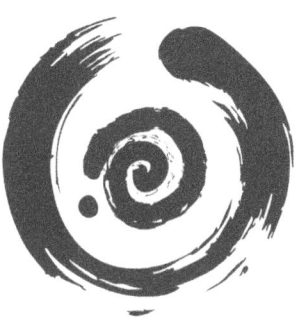

Kiotsukete
Learn to Take Care

Journal Prompts for Chapter 4.
Kiotsukete – Learn to Take Care

1. **Self-Trust Reflection:**
   When was the last time I truly trusted my intuition or inner voice? What was the outcome?

2. **Daily Self-Care:**
   What is one small, meaningful act of care I can do for myself each day this week?

3. **Nature Connection:**
   How do I feel after spending time in nature? How can I make this a regular part of my wellness routine?

4. **Food as Care:**
   Do my eating habits reflect care and respect for my body? Where might I make small, nourishing changes?

5. **Boundaries and Energy:**

   Where in my life do I need to say "no" more often to protect my energy and wellbeing?

6. **Joy Inventory:**

   What activities, people, or places bring me joy? How can I invite more of this joy into my everyday life?

7. **Rest Check-In:**

   Am I getting enough rest—physically, mentally, and emotionally? If not, what might I change?

8. **Relationships and Support:**

   Who are the people I feel most supported by? How can I nurture those relationships?

9. **Movement Reframe:**

   How can I move my body in ways that feel joyful and healing rather than forced or routine?

10. **Ritual of Care:**

    What would my ideal daily self-care routine look like if time, money, or guilt weren't barriers?

五

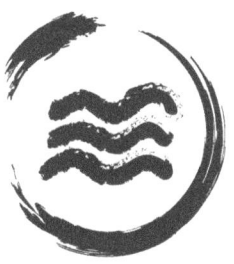

Ganbatte
Always Do Your Best by Hanging In There

Journal Prompts: Chapter 5. Ganbatte – Always Do Your Best by Hanging in There

1. **Embracing the Struggle:**
   Think of a recent challenge you've faced. How did it shape you? What did you learn about yourself during that struggle?

2. **Giving Your All:**
   When was the last time you gave your absolute best effort toward something? How did it feel, and what was the outcome?

3. **Time and Commitment:**
   Are there any areas of your life where you feel you could be more punctual or committed? How would showing up on time impact your overall sense of purpose?

4. **Authenticity Check:**

   When was the last time you felt fully yourself—authentic and unapologetic? How can you bring more of your true self into your daily actions?

5. **Supporting Others:**

   Think of someone in your life who might be struggling. How can you show up for them, and what small act of kindness could you offer today?

6. **Honesty and Integrity:**

   Is there an area of your life where you feel out of alignment with your values or truth? What would it take for you to be more honest in that area?

7. **Staying the Course:**

   What is a long-term goal you've set for yourself? How can you remind yourself to stay focused and committed during the challenging moments of that journey?

8. **Celebrating Progress:**

   Reflect on a time when you didn't give up on something. Even if it wasn't perfect, what positive changes or lessons did you gain from sticking with it?

9. **Learning from Failure:**

   Have you ever experienced a failure that, in hindsight, was actually a stepping stone to something better? How did you overcome the fear of failure, and what did it teach you?

10. **Resilience in Action:**

    What personal qualities or habits do you rely on to help you stay resilient when times get tough? How can you cultivate these qualities even further?

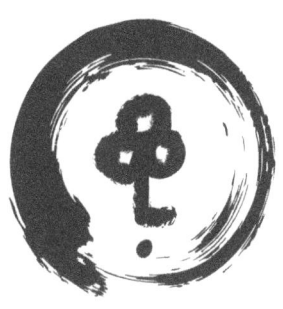

Kaizen
Continuously Improve

Journal Prompts for Chapter 6.
Kaizen – Continuously Improve

1. **Reflect on Your Current Growth**
   How have you made progress in your life, work, or personal development over the last year? What small changes have you made that have resulted in noticeable improvements?

2. **Identify Areas for Improvement**
   What areas of your life (e.g., health, relationships, career, personal growth) do you feel could benefit from small, continuous improvements? Write about the first step you can take to begin this process.

3. **The Power of Small Changes**
   Think of a time when a small change led to big results. What was the change, and how did it affect your life in

the long term? How can you apply this lesson to other areas of your life?

4. **Overcoming Obstacles to Improvement**
   What are the obstacles or challenges that hold you back from continuous improvement? How can you reframe or approach these challenges in a way that helps you grow despite them?

5. **Consistency vs. Perfection**
   Reflect on the difference between striving for perfection and focusing on consistent improvement. How can embracing imperfection help you make consistent progress toward your goals?

6. **Self-Reflection on the Kaizen Mindset**
   What does the Kaizen mindset (continuous improvement) mean to you? How can you incorporate it into your daily life and mindset to become a better version of yourself over time?

7. **Goal Setting with Kaizen**
   Set a small, actionable goal for yourself based on the Kaizen principle. Break it down into micro-steps that you can take every day. What's the first step you'll take to work toward this goal?

8. **Celebrating Small Wins**
   Write about a small victory you've experienced recently. How did it contribute to your personal growth? Why is it important to acknowledge and celebrate small wins?

9. **Continuous Learning**
   How can you integrate learning into your everyday routine? What are some skills or topics you'd like to learn more about, and how can small, consistent actions help you improve over time?

10. **Long-Term Vision**

Looking ahead, where do you see yourself in one year if you practice Kaizen, continuous improvement in all areas of your life? What will your progress look like, and how will it feel?

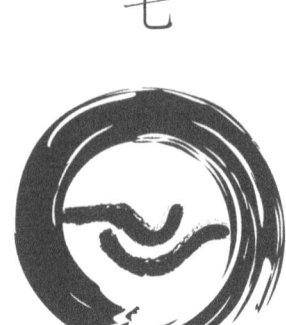

Shikata ga nai
Accept What Cannot Be Helped

Journal Prompts for Chapter 7. Shikata ga nai – Accept What Cannot Be Helped

1. **Acceptance of the Uncontrollable**
   Reflect on a situation in your life that you cannot change. How does accepting this reality, rather than resisting it, make you feel? What steps can you take to find peace with this situation?

2. **Learning to Let Go**
   Think about something you've been holding onto emotionally or mentally that you know you can't change. What would it feel like to let go of this burden, and how might your life improve if you did?

3. **Meditation and Acceptance**
   Have you ever used meditation to come to terms with something you couldn't change? Write about an experience where meditation helped you release

control or come to a place of peace with what was out of your hands.

4. **Shifting Perspectives**

Think of a difficult situation in your life. How can you change your perspective to see it in a more positive light or find a lesson in it? What new angle can you take that allows you to accept it?

5. **Embracing Life's Imperfections**

How does the idea of embracing imperfection resonate with you? Write about a time when embracing something imperfect brought you peace or helped you move forward.

6. **Resilience Through Acceptance**

Reflect on a time when you were faced with something difficult to accept. How did you manage to stay resilient during this time? How did acceptance play a role in your ability to navigate it?

7. **Healing Through Acceptance**

Write about something in your life that requires healing. What steps can you take to move toward healing, and how can acceptance be part of that process?

8. **Self-Compassion in the Face of What Cannot Be Changed**

Are there any areas where you're hard on yourself because you're unable to change certain circumstances? How can you practice self-compassion instead of self-criticism in those moments?

9. **Gratitude for What Remains**

After reflecting on something you can't change, what are you grateful for in your life that you still have control over? Write a gratitude list for the things that are still within your grasp.

10. **Moving Forward After Acceptance**

How can you take positive steps forward after accepting something that cannot be changed? What actions can you take to grow from this experience, and how can you move forward with a lighter heart?

11. **The Role of Supportive People**

How do the people around you help you when you are struggling to accept something you cannot change? Reflect on the impact of support from others in helping you accept and move on.

12. **Forest Bathing and Acceptance**

Have you ever practiced forest bathing or immersing yourself in nature to help you accept things beyond your control? Describe how nature might help you shift your mindset and bring acceptance into your life.

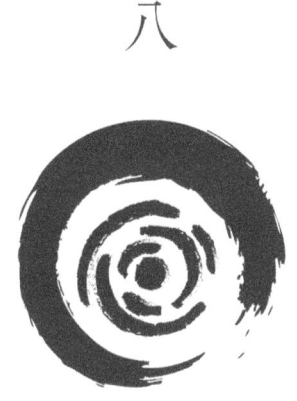

Yumaru
Care for Your Inner Circle

Journal Prompts for Chapter 8. Yumaru – Care for Your Inner Circle

1. **Defining Your Inner Circle**
   Who are the people you consider part of your inner circle? Reflect on the qualities that make these relationships special and valuable to you. What do these people bring into your life that you can't find elsewhere?

2. **The Importance of Community**
   How has being part of a community (whether family, friends, or a larger group) impacted your life? Write about the positive effects of connection and support from others, and how it nurtures your well-being.

3. **Show, Don't Tell**

   Reflect on a recent situation where you expressed care or love for someone in your inner circle. Did you show your feelings through actions, or were they expressed in words? How can you deepen your connections through thoughtful actions instead of just words?

4. **Being Present in Relationships**

   Think about a time when you were truly present with someone, free from distractions and fully engaged in the moment. How did that moment strengthen your bond? What might change in your relationships if you were more present going forward?

5. **Offering Support Without Expectations**

   Write about a time when you helped someone without expecting anything in return. How did it feel to give without anticipation of reciprocation? How can you practice offering more of this kind of support in your relationships?

6. **Proactive Care in Your Circle**

   How can you take the initiative in your relationships? Think about small, proactive steps you can take to show your love, care, and support for the people around you. What's one thing you can do today to strengthen your inner circle?

7. **Being Thoughtful in Your Relationships**

   Reflect on the last time someone did something thoughtful for you. How did it make you feel? How can you show thoughtfulness to the people in your inner circle, and what simple actions would have the most positive impact on them?

8. **The Value of Vulnerability**

Vulnerability can deepen relationships. Write about a time when you allowed yourself to be vulnerable with someone in your inner circle. What was the outcome, and how did it affect your relationship with that person?

9. **Balancing Giving and Receiving**

Consider how balanced your relationships are in terms of giving and receiving. Do you feel that both you and those in your inner circle offer support to one another? How can you ensure that you are giving enough, but also allowing yourself to receive support?

10. **Building a Stronger Inner Circle**

How can you strengthen the connections in your inner circle? Reflect on what you might need to do to nurture these relationships, whether through communication, spending quality time together, or other meaningful ways.

11. **The Power of Active Listening**

Reflect on the last conversation you had with someone close to you. Did you truly listen to them, or were you more focused on what you were going to say next? How can active listening improve your relationships and show that you truly care?

12. **Creating a Culture of Care**

How can you cultivate a culture of care within your inner circle? Consider what actions, behaviours, or attitudes you could encourage that would help everyone feel supported, valued, and loved. What can you do to set an example of care?

13. **When to Let Go**

   Sometimes, we need to let go of people who no longer align with our values or well-being. Write about a time when you had to distance yourself from someone. What did you learn from that experience, and how did it impact your inner circle?

14. **Gratitude for Your Inner Circle**

   Take a moment to express gratitude for the people in your inner circle. What are the specific ways in which they enrich your life? Write a thank-you letter to someone in your inner circle who has supported you and made a difference in your life.

九

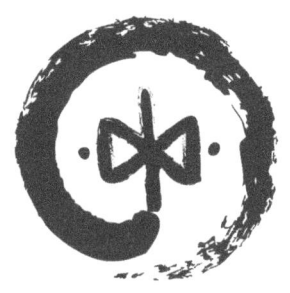

Kansha
Cultivate Sincere Gratitude

Journal Prompts for Chapter 9. Kansha – Cultivate Sincere Gratitude

1. **What are three things you are genuinely grateful for today?**
   Reflect on the small moments, people, or experiences that made you feel thankful today. Write down what they are and why they stand out to you.

2. **How can you practice gratitude more authentically in your daily life?**
   Think about areas in your life where you may express gratitude out of habit rather than genuine feeling. How can you make your gratitude more heartfelt and sincere?

3. **In what ways does gratitude improve your perspective when you face challenges?**
Write about a difficult situation you've experienced recently. How did practicing gratitude shift your mindset or help you cope with the situation?

4. **What is something positive that happened in your life recently, no matter how small, that you often overlook?**
Focus on a moment you might have taken for granted. How can you bring more appreciation to these smaller, everyday blessings?

5. **Who is someone in your life that you would like to express more gratitude towards, and why?**
Write a letter (even if you don't send it) to someone you feel you need to thank. Express why they matter to you and the ways they've impacted your life.

6. **How does being grateful for the present moment change your relationship with time?**
Reflect on how focusing on the present, rather than always striving for the future, changes how you experience time. Do you feel more grounded when you practice gratitude in the now?

7. **How does the act of expressing gratitude affect your emotional well-being?**
Explore how expressing gratitude makes you feel. Do you notice changes in your mood, stress levels, or sense of peace after practicing gratitude?

8. **What personal strengths or qualities can you express gratitude for in yourself?**
Write about the qualities that make you unique and how they have helped you in different aspects of your

life. Why is it important to appreciate and nurture your own strengths?

9. **How can you show appreciation for the people who may not expect it, but truly deserve it?**
Reflect on those who quietly support or positively influence your life. How can you express your gratitude to them, even if they don't ask for it?

10. **What are some simple actions you can take to cultivate gratitude in others?**
Think of ways to spread gratitude to the people around you, whether through a kind word, an act of service, or a heartfelt thank-you. What impact do you think this could have on your relationships?

11. **What is one challenge in your life right now that could be reframed through gratitude?**
Consider a current struggle or challenge and think about how you could shift your perspective to see the lessons or growth opportunities it brings. How does gratitude alter your view of this challenge?

12. **How can you use gratitude as a tool for healing?**
Write about a time in your life when practicing gratitude helped you heal emotionally or physically. How did it contribute to your recovery or growth?

13. **In what ways can you make gratitude a consistent part of your day?**
Consider simple daily habits that you can adopt to regularly practice gratitude, whether through journaling, meditation, or other rituals. How can you integrate this practice to make it a natural part of your routine?

14. **How does sincere gratitude improve your connection to others?**

Reflect on how expressing authentic gratitude has affected your relationships. Have you noticed it strengthening bonds or creating more openness with others?

15. **What role does gratitude play in helping you live a more peaceful, fulfilled life?**

Write about the connection between gratitude and inner peace. How does a consistent practice of gratitude contribute to your overall sense of well-being and contentment?

These prompts are designed to help you explore the deep and transformative power of gratitude in your life, guiding you toward a mindset of appreciation that can create meaningful change.

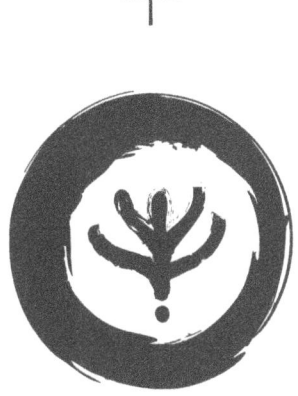

Osettai
Be of Service to Others

Journal Prompts Chapter 10.
Embracing the Spirit of Osettai

1. **When was the last time I gave something to someone without expecting anything in return? How did it make me feel?**
   (Reflect on moments of pure generosity or kindness, no matter how small.)

2. **What are some small, thoughtful ways I can practice Osettai in my everyday life?**
   (Think about actions like offering help, making tea, writing a kind note, or sharing a skill.)

3. **How do I respond when I receive kindness or help? Do I allow myself to receive fully?**
   (Osettai is about both giving and receiving, explore how you honour both sides.)

4. **Who in my life might need a gesture of unexpected kindness right now? What could I offer them?**

   (This could be time, attention, encouragement, or a thoughtful gift.)

5. **How can I bring more warmth and sincerity into my interactions with strangers?**

   (Consider how simple gestures, like a smile, eye contact, or patience can embody Osettai.)

6. **In what ways have I benefitted from the kindness of others that I didn't see coming?**

   (Write about a time when someone's selfless gesture uplifted or surprised you.)

7. **What holds me back from giving freely? How can I let go of that resistance?**

   (Explore fears around scarcity, worthiness, or time that might prevent you from giving.)

8. **How does practicing Osettai connect me to a larger sense of purpose or community?**

   (Reflect on how giving creates bonds and a sense of shared humanity.)

9. **How would my daily life shift if I approached each person I met with a mindset of service and presence?**

   (Imagine your relationships, work, and home life with this principle guiding you.)

10. **Create a "Kindness Plan" for this week, what will you do, for whom, and how will you remain unattached to the outcome?**

    (Use this as a practical way to embody Osettai intentionally.)

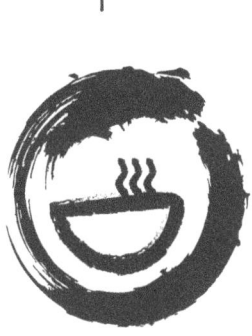

Chado
The Pleasures of Matcha and the Japanese Tea Culture

Journal Prompts for Chapter 11. The Pleasures of Matcha and the Japanese Tea Culture

1. **Reflect on Your First Encounter with Tea or a Tea Ceremony**
   - What was your initial impression of tea, especially matcha?
   - How did your understanding or appreciation of tea evolve over time?

2. **Mindfulness in the Tea Ceremony**
   - Think about the process of making tea, what aspects of the ceremony help you slow down and become present?
   - How can you incorporate more mindful moments like this into your daily routine?

3. **The Ritual of Tea Making**
   - Reflect on the idea of ritual in your life. Are there small rituals you practice that bring calm or clarity?

o How might you create a personal tea ceremony that helps centre you during stressful moments?

4. **Matcha and Your Health**
   o How do you feel after drinking matcha or green tea?
   o Have you noticed any health benefits from incorporating it into your life (increased focus, improved energy, etc.)?

5. **Hospitality and Sharing**
   o In Japanese culture, offering tea is a sign of hospitality. Think of a time when you welcomed someone with warmth and care.
   o How can you make moments of hospitality more intentional in your own life?

6. **The Beauty of Imperfection in the Tea Ceremony**
   o Reflect on the idea of imperfection within the tea ceremony and the grace it represents.
   o How can you embrace imperfections in your own life, allowing them to bring beauty rather than frustration?

7. **Personal Peace Through Rituals**
   o How does the act of brewing matcha or participating in a tea ceremony help you find inner peace?
   o What other small rituals or activities help you experience peace or clarity?

8. **Connecting with Tradition**
   o Tea ceremonies have been passed down through generations in Japan. How does participating in a practice with such rich tradition make you feel connected to a larger community or history?
   o Are there traditions or rituals in your own culture that bring you comfort and connection?

9. **Create Your Own Tea Ceremony**
   - Imagine your ideal tea ceremony, what elements would be included?
   - How can you create a peaceful tea ritual in your daily life?

10. **The Role of Gratitude in the Ceremony**

- In the tea ceremony, each action is filled with intention and respect. How can you bring this level of intention into your daily practices?
- What aspects of your life do you feel most grateful for, and how can you express that gratitude more often?

十二

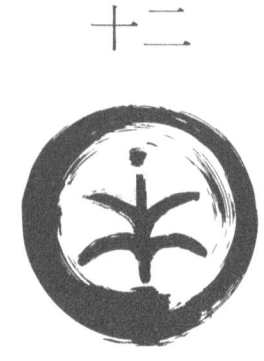

Ikebana
The Art of Flower Arranging

Journal Prompts for Chapter 12: Ikebana - The Art of Flower Arranging:

1. **Reflect on Nature's Beauty**
   Take a moment to observe the natural world around you. What do you notice about the imperfections and unique qualities of plants, flowers, and trees? How can you apply these observations to your Ikebana practice or other areas of your life?

2. **The Role of Imperfection**
   Ikebana celebrates the "perfect imperfection" of nature. How do you feel about imperfections in your own life? How can embracing imperfection help you find beauty and peace in daily life?

3. **Mindfulness in Flower Arranging**
   How does the act of flower arranging or being creative with nature help you practice mindfulness? How do

you feel before, during, and after creating an Ikebana arrangement? What emotions arise during the process?

4. **Balance and Harmony**

   In Ikebana, balance is key. How can you apply the principles of balance and harmony from Ikebana to your own life? Are there areas in your life that feel out of balance, and how can you realign them?

5. **Personal Connection to Flowers**

   What does working with flowers or plants mean to you? Do you have a personal connection to any specific flower, colour, or plant? Why does it resonate with you?

6. **Creating with Intention**

   Ikebana is about creating with purpose. When you create something, whether it's an arrangement, a piece of art, or any project—what intention do you bring to it? What values do you want to express through your creativity?

7. **The Art of Simplicity**

   Ikebana emphasizes simplicity and space. How can you simplify different areas of your life to create more space for peace and clarity? What are the things you can let go of that no longer serve you?

8. **Reflection on Growth and Change**

   Ikebana is rooted in the transient nature of life and the changing seasons. How do you personally experience growth and change? What can you learn from the natural cycles of growth, blooming, and fading?

9. **Connecting with Your Inner Self**

   How does the act of arranging flowers help you connect with your inner self? How do you feel when you work with natural elements? What might this practice teach you about your emotional or spiritual life?

10. **Exploring Creativity**

How does creating something from nature, whether through Ikebana or other forms of art—help you explore your creativity? What role does creativity play in your daily life, and how can you nurture it more often?

These journal prompts are designed to help you reflect deeply on the philosophical and personal aspects of Ikebana, enriching both your practice and your understanding of this beautiful Japanese art.

十三

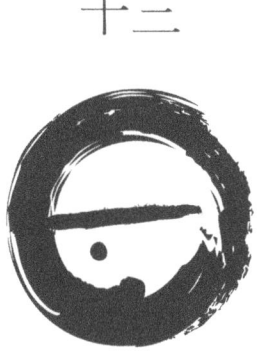

Kanso
Embracing Simplicity Through Decluttering

Journal prompts for Chapter 13. *Kanso* and the importance of decluttering:

1. **How does clutter affect your emotional and mental state?**
   Take a moment to reflect on how you feel when you're surrounded by clutter. Do you notice feelings of stress, anxiety, or distraction? How does your space influence your mood or productivity?

2. **What is your relationship with possessions?**
   Reflect on your connection with the objects you own. Do any of them hold sentimental value or bring you joy? Are there items that you're holding onto simply because of habit or societal expectations?

3. **What areas of your home feel most cluttered or chaotic?**
   Consider the areas of your home that tend to accumulate clutter. What spaces do you find yourself avoiding or

feeling overwhelmed by? What might it feel like to simplify or reorganize these areas?

4. **What does simplicity look like to you?**

   Visualize your ideal living space. What does it look like? How does it make you feel? How can you create an environment that reflects simplicity, calm, and balance?

5. **What items in your home truly serve a purpose or bring you joy?**

   Take a moment to go through the items in your space and evaluate them. Which ones do you use regularly or find meaningful? Which ones have lost their significance or no longer serve a useful purpose?

6. **How do you practice mindfulness when it comes to your possessions?**

   How aware are you when acquiring new items for your home? Are you choosing things intentionally, or are you collecting out of habit? Consider how you might practice mindfulness in your purchasing and organizing habits.

7. **What emotions arise when you think about decluttering?**

   Decluttering can be an emotional process. What feelings arise when you think about letting go of possessions? Are there any items that are particularly hard to part with? Why?

8. **How does the idea of "creating space for peace" resonate with you?**

   Reflect on the notion that decluttering isn't just about cleaning—it's about creating mental and emotional space. How can removing excess physical clutter help to clear mental clutter in your life?

9. **What steps can you take today to start embracing** *Kanso* **in your home?**

   What small action can you take right now to move toward a simpler, more organized space? Whether it's sorting through one drawer, setting aside time for decluttering, or simply letting go of an item, what can you do today to bring simplicity into your life?

10. **How does your environment impact your well-being?**

    Consider how the space around you affects your overall health and happiness. How do cluttered, disorganized spaces impact your mental and emotional well-being? How might adopting *Kanso* improve your lifestyle?

These prompts can guide you in reflecting on the principles of *Kanso* and how you can apply them to your life, helping you embrace a simpler, more intentional way of living.

十四

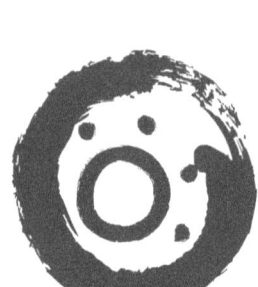

Ikigai
The Japanese Secret to a Fulfilling Life

Journal Prompts for Chapter 14: Ikigai

1. **What gets you out of bed in the morning?**
   Reflect on the activities or thoughts that make you feel excited, alive, or at peace. What do they reveal about your ikigai?

2. **List three moments from your life when you felt deeply fulfilled.**
   What were you doing? Who were you with? What values or passions were being expressed?

3. **What are your core values?**
   Write down 3–5 values that are most important to you. How do these guide your daily actions?

4. **What do you love doing so much that you lose track of time?**
   Explore activities that bring you into a state of flow. These are strong clues to your ikigai.

5. **What are you good at?**
   Identify your natural talents or skills you've developed over time. How do you enjoy using them?

6. **What does the world need that you care about?**
   Think about causes or issues that matter to you. Where could you make a meaningful contribution?

7. **What can you be paid for that aligns with your passion and strengths?**
   Consider your current or ideal work. Does it align with your sense of purpose or ikigai?

8. **How can you bring more purpose into your everyday routine?**
   What small changes or habits could you adopt to feel more connected to your ikigai daily?

9. **Who inspires you with their sense of purpose?**
   Reflect on someone who lives with clear direction and passion. What can you learn from them?

10. **What would you do if money and expectations were no object?**
    Allow yourself to dream. What does this version of your life look like?

These prompts are designed to guide readers inward, helping them discover their personal ikigai and align more of their lives with it.

十五

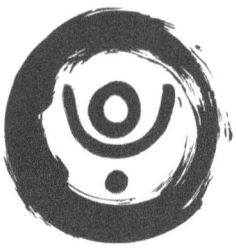

Meiso
Japanese Styles of Meditation and the Science of Stillness

Journal Prompts for Chapter 15:
Japanese Meditation Practices

1. **What does meditation mean to you right now?**
   How do you perceive stillness and mindfulness in your current lifestyle? Has that changed over time?

2. **Have you ever practiced any form of meditation?**
   Reflect on your experience. What helped you feel grounded or centred? What challenged you?

3. **What type of meditation practice resonates with you most—Zazen (Zen sitting), Kinhin (walking meditation), or Shikantaza ("just sitting")? Why?**
   Explore which Japanese meditation style feels most approachable and meaningful for your life.

4. **When was the last time you sat in silence without distraction?**
   What did you notice in your body, mind, and emotions during that time?

5. **What role does breathe play in your daily life?**
   Try focusing on your breathing for just 2 minutes. How did that feel? Could this become a micro-meditation practice for you?

6. **What does "being present" look like in your daily activities?**
   Are their areas in your life where you operate on autopilot? How might you bring more mindfulness into them?

7. **What distractions keep you from connecting with stillness?**
   Make a list of external (e.g., noise, technology) and internal (e.g., stress, overthinking) distractions. Which one can you gently reduce this week?

8. **How do you currently manage stress?**
   Could a simple daily meditation practice support you in regulating your nervous system?

9. **What are three benefits you imagine or have experienced from practicing mindfulness or meditation?**
   Consider the emotional, physical, or cognitive shifts that may happen with consistent stillness.

10. **How can you create a personal meditation corner or routine inspired by Japanese simplicity (Kanso) and calm?**
    What would make this space feel peaceful, intentional, and yours?

These prompts aim to help readers explore their own connection to Japanese meditation traditions and uncover practical ways to create inner calm and clarity.

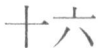

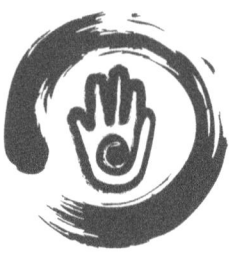

Dento Ryoho
Traditional Japanese Healing Practices
History, Science & Modern Adaptations

Journal Prompts – Chapter 16: Traditional Japanese Healing Practices

1. **Which traditional Japanese healing practice resonated with you the most and why?**
   (Was it Reiki, forest bathing, onsen bathing, Kampo medicine, or another practice?)

2. **Have you ever experienced a healing moment in nature? Describe it.**
   (What were you doing, what did you feel, and how did it affect your body or mind?)

3. **How do you currently support your own healing— physically, emotionally, and spiritually?**
   (What could you integrate from the Japanese healing philosophy into your routine?)

4. **If you could design a weekly healing ritual for yourself based on Japanese traditions, what would it include?**

   (A hot bath with hinoki oil? A walk in nature? A tea ceremony? A Reiki session?)

5. **Explore your beliefs around energy and wellness.**

   (Do you believe in energetic healing like Reiki or shiatsu? How open are you to subtle energy practices?)

6. **Reflect on the idea that healing is both preventative and intuitive.**

   (What would change in your life if you saw healing as a daily rhythm instead of a reaction to illness?)

7. **Write about a time when slowing down felt deeply healing.**

   (What allowed you to slow down, and what impact did it have on your health or mindset?)

8. **Which healing elements from Japanese culture could enhance your home environment?**

   (Think about scents, textures, natural materials, or even sounds like wind chimes or water features.)

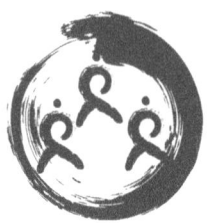

Kyōdōtai and Kizuna
The Power of Community and Connection in Japanese Culture

Journal Prompts – Chapter 17: Kyodotai & Kizuna - Community & Connection

1. **Reflect on your sense of community.**
   Who are the people in your life you feel most connected to? What makes those relationships meaningful to you?

2. **Where do you experience *kyōdōtai*?**
   Think about a group you belong to (family, workplace, neighbourhood, online community). How does it reflect shared values or responsibilities?

3. **Describe a time you felt deep *kizuna* (emotional bond) with someone.**
   What created that connection? How did it support your emotional or physical wellbeing?

4. **Explore your *tsunagari* (links) with the wider world.**
   How do you stay connected to people you don't see every day? What helps you feel linked to others, even at a distance?

5. **Do you feel a stronger sense of connection in in-person or digital communities? Why?**

   What qualities make a space (online or offline) feel safe and supportive to you?

6. **What small gesture can you do this week to strengthen a bond or build community?**

   Think about a note, act of kindness, or shared activity you could offer.

7. **What does "belonging" mean to you?**

   Do you feel a sense of belonging in your daily life? If not, what would help you cultivate it?

8. **Imagine your ideal community.**

   What values would it be based on? How would people support and connect with one another?

十八

Kintsugi
Embracing Imperfection and Finding Beauty in the Broken

Journal Prompts: Chapter 18. Kintsugi – The Art of Healing and Wholeness

1. **What parts of my life or self, have felt broken—and how have I begun to mend them?**
   (Reflect on personal challenges and your healing journey.)

2. **Where in my life can I apply the Kintsugi mindset—honouring scars instead of hiding them?**
   (Think emotionally, physically, spiritually, or even in relationships.)

3. **What golden lessons have emerged from my struggles or setbacks?**
   (Identify the wisdom that came from difficult experiences.)

4. **If I could "fill the cracks" of my past with gold, what would that gold represent?**
   (Write about values like resilience, compassion, or strength.)

5. **In what ways have my perceived imperfections made me more human—or more beautiful?**

   (Explore the idea that our flaws make us unique and lovable.)

6. **Who in my life models the spirit of Kintsugi— someone who carries their healing with grace?**

   (What have you learned from them?)

7. **What relationships or memories do I wish to repair with gentleness and care?**

   (Consider what needs mending, not discarding.)

8. **What daily or creative rituals help me reconnect with my sense of wholeness?**

   (Think about writing, art, meditation, movement, etc.)

9. **If I were to create a symbolic Kintsugi piece from my life, what would it be?**

   (Describe the object, the cracks, and the gold you'd use to repair it.)

10. **What does it mean to me to be "whole," even if I am not perfect?**

    (Define wholeness in your own words.)

These prompts invite reflection, healing, and celebration of your beautifully mended self.

十九

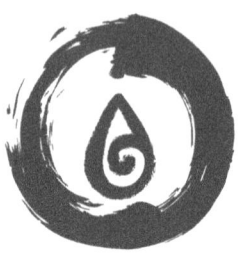

The Longevity Science of Ofuro
The Sacred Japanese Bathing Tradition

Journal Prompts: Chapter 19. Embracing Ofuro for Wellness and Reflection

1. **How does taking a warm bath or shower help me physically and emotionally unwind?**
   (Describe the sensations, emotions, or thoughts that surface during or after.)

2. **When was the last time I fully allowed myself to slow down and relax without distraction?**
   (Explore the obstacles to relaxation and how you might overcome them.)

3. **What elements make my bathing ritual feel sacred or restorative?**
   (Think about water temperature, lighting, scents, silence, or music.)

4. **What would it look like to turn my daily hygiene routine into a ritual of self-love?**
   (Imagine a calm, intentional version of your bath or shower time.)

5. **What am I ready to wash away—physically, mentally, or emotionally?**
   (Let the metaphor of cleansing guide your inner release.)

6. **How can I carry the stillness and calm of ofuro into the rest of my day or evening?**
   (Write about habits or boundaries that help extend that peaceful state.)

7. **Are there any scents or ingredients (e.g., yuzu, hinoki, green tea) I associate with peace or healing? Why?**
   (Explore how sensory details impact your mood and memory.)

8. **What does the concept of "purification" mean to me—beyond the physical?**
   (Reflect on how rituals like ofuro can support spiritual or emotional clarity.)

9. **How can I create space in my life for quiet rituals like ofuro, even when I'm busy?**
   (Get practical about protecting time for wellness and solitude.)

10. **What intention do I want to set the next time I immerse myself in water?**
    (Choose a word, feeling, or mantra to hold during your next bath or shower.)

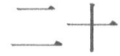

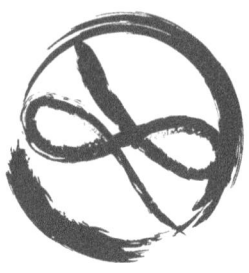

Shodo
The Way of Writing

Journal Prompts: Chapter 20.
Shodō – The Way of Writing

1. **What emotions arise when I slow down and focus on each stroke or word I write?**

   (Consider how mindful writing feels in your body and mind.)

2. **How does writing by hand change the way I express myself compared to typing?**

   (Reflect on the tactile, intentional process of putting pen to paper.)

3. **What word or phrase holds deep meaning for me right now?**

   (Choose one and explore its significance — you could even try drawing it in your own style.)

4. **Where in my life do I need more *flow* and less perfection?**
   (Calligraphy embraces fluid motion and imperfection — how does this idea apply to your life?)

5. **If I could express a feeling or memory through a single brushstroke, what would it be?**
   (Let your imagination interpret the emotions you carry.)

6. **What does "presence" mean to me, and how can I cultivate it through creative practices like Shodō?**
   (Explore the connection between creativity and mindfulness.)

7. **What does my handwriting say about me today? How has it changed over time?**
   (Your script can be a mirror of your inner state, observe without judgment.)

8. **How can I use writing as a meditative practice in my daily routine?**
   (Journaling, gratitude lists, letters, poetry, mantras?)

9. **What lessons can I learn from Japanese calligraphy's emphasis on simplicity, elegance, and intention?**
   (Reflect on how these values might shape your lifestyle.)

10. **If I wrote a letter of gratitude today, who would I send it to — and what would I say?**
    (Use this as an opportunity to combine Shodō with Osettai acts of kindness.)

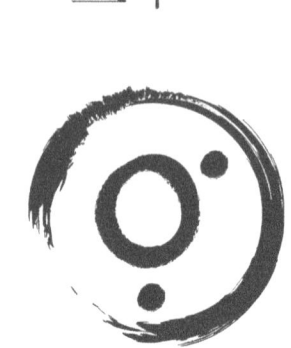

Ichigo Ichie
Once in a lifetime encounter

Journal Prompts: Chapter 21. *Ichigo Ichie* – One Time, One Encounter

1. **Describe a moment from today that felt truly unique or meaningful.**
   (Why did it stand out? What emotions did it stir in you?)

2. **When was the last time you felt completely present with someone?**
   (What made that moment feel special? Would you change anything about how you showed up?)

3. **How would you act differently if you knew this very moment would never come again?**
   (Reflect on how impermanence can bring deeper presence.)

4. **Write about a recent encounter — even if it was brief — that left a lasting impression.**
   (What made it memorable? What did you learn from it?)

5. **What is one small, everyday ritual you can approach with full presence and appreciation?**
   (Tea drinking, walking, brushing your hair, watching the sunset?)

6. **Think of someone you see often — how can you connect with them today as if for the first (and only) time?**
   (Explore how Ichigo Ichie can deepen your relationships.)

7. **What past moment do you now realize was an *Ichigo Ichie* moment?**
   (Why is it only now that you recognize its uniqueness?)

8. **What helps you stay in the present? What tends to pull you away?**
   (Be honest about your habits and distractions.)

9. **Write a message to your future self about what you're experiencing right now.**
   (Capture this moment, the sights, feelings, thoughts as a one-time gift.)

10. **How can you bring the spirit of *Ichigo Ichie* into your work, your meals, or your conversations today?**
    (Set an intention and observe how it transforms your day.)

二十二

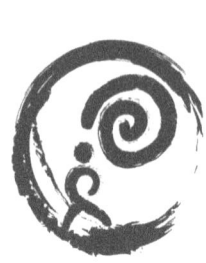

The Art of Japanese
Skincare & Wellness

Journal Prompts: Chapter 22. Japanese Beauty Rituals – Graceful, Natural, Mindful

1. **What does "beauty" mean to you beyond appearance?**

   (How do you define beauty from a holistic or wellness perspective?)

2. **How does your current skincare or self-care routine make you feel emotionally and physically?**

   (Are there any rituals you want to introduce or refine?)

3. **Have you ever practiced skincare as a meditative ritual rather than a routine?**

   (Describe what that experience was like or how you could make your rituals more intentional.)

4. **Japanese beauty places emphasis on simplicity and consistency. What steps can you simplify in your routine to bring more calm and balance?**

5. **How do you nourish your skin from the inside out?**
   (Reflect on your hydration, nutrition, and stress levels and how they affect your skin.)
6. **Write about a moment when you felt truly radiant— what was contributing to that glow?**
7. **Are there areas of your body or appearance you've been overly critical of?**
   (How can you shift to gratitude for all that your body does for you?)
8. **Japanese rituals often use natural elements like green tea, rice water, seaweed, and camellia oil. Which of these ingredients or traditions are you curious to try, and why?**
9. **How might embracing aging as a beautiful, graceful process shift the way you approach your skincare and wellness practices?**
10. **Create an affirmation that aligns with how you want to feel in your skin every day.**
    (Examples: "I glow from inner peace," or "My skin reflects my care and joy.")

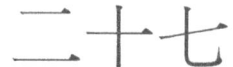

二十七

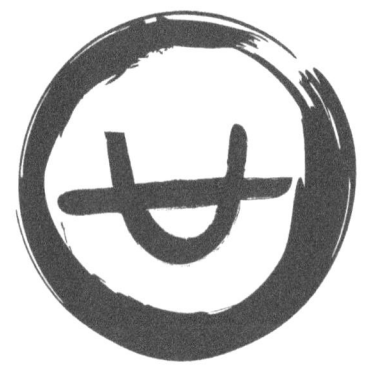

Japanese Recipes

Barbara's Favourite Japanese, Easy to cook Recipes

Introduction

When I moved to Japan, I never imagined how deeply the culture, especially its food, would transform my life. What began as a curiosity soon became a daily ritual: preparing simple, seasonal meals rooted in balance, beauty, and nourishment. Over the years I lived there, I embraced not just the flavours of Japanese cuisine, but also the deeper philosophy it embodies, one of respect for ingredients, mindful preparation, and the power of food to heal and connect.

These recipes are a heartfelt collection of the dishes I learned, loved, and lived by. Recipes I cooked daily in my home in Japan, and many of which I still include in my weekly meal plans for their extraordinary health benefits. Whether it's the gut-friendly goodness of miso soup, the antioxidant-rich matcha, or the calming rhythm of preparing tamagoyaki, these meals have taught me that food can be both nourishing and restorative.

Japanese cuisine is grounded in the principles of *eiyōshoku* (nutrient-rich food), seasonal eating, and a gentle, deliberate approach to cooking. Modern science continues to validate these traditions: fermented foods like miso and natto support gut health, sea vegetables offer essential minerals, and dishes rich in umami enhance satisfaction without excess salt or fat. It's no wonder that Japan has one of the highest life expectancies in the world.

But Japanese food is more than nutrition. It is also a cultural experience. Before every meal, we say "Itadakimasu", a humble expression of gratitude meaning *"I humbly receive."* It's a reminder to honour the hands that grew, harvested, and prepared the food. And at the end of each meal, we say "Gochisōsama deshita," meaning *"Thank you for the feast,"* to acknowledge the joy and effort behind it.

My hope is that these recipes invite you not only to eat well but to live well. Cook them slowly. Savour them fully. Let them bring presence, pleasure, and nourishment into your life, one bowl, one bite, one beautiful ritual at a time.

With warmth and wellness,
Barbara
Itadakimasu!

Nourishing Our Bodies with Delicious Japanese Food

You might be curious as to why this chapter doesn't immediately follow Chapter 3, Eiyoshoku. The reason is that it's intended as an additional prompt to reassess your dietary habits. While you may have already started incorporating some Japanese ingredients, fully embracing them might have been challenging.

This chapter is designed to provide the momentum you need to delve deeper into your meals, seeking nourishment and balance.

In Japan, food isn't just about sustenance; it's a way of life, a cultural experience that is deeply tied to wellness, mindfulness, and balance. Over the years, I've come to appreciate the Japanese approach to food, not only for its rich variety and exquisite flavours but also for the way it nurtures both the body and the spirit. In this chapter, I'll share with you some principles of the Japanese diet that you can incorporate into your own life for greater health and well-being. Don't worry if you can't implement them all at once, take it slow, and over time, you'll notice the incredible benefits.

1. **Drink Plenty of Water and Green Tea**
   In Japan, hydration is key to maintaining health. You'll often see people sipping water or green tea throughout the day, especially green tea, which is an integral part of Japanese culture. Drinking water is a simple but essential way to maintain hydration, flush out toxins, and support digestion. Traditional Japanese tea culture places a strong emphasis on green tea, which is rich in antioxidants, particularly catechins, that have been shown to support heart health, boost metabolism, and protect against illnesses. Aim to drink at least 2 litres of water a day and incorporate green tea into your routine. If you're feeling adventurous, try a Japanese tea like matcha, which is ground green tea leaves that provide an extra boost of antioxidants.

2. **Eat Plenty of Fresh Fruits and Vegetables**

Japanese cuisine is built around a variety of seasonal fruits and vegetables, often in their freshest, most natural form. From daikon radish to edamame, shiso leaves, ginger, and nori, Japanese meals are filled with fresh, nutrient-dense produce. In Japan, it's common to consume a wide variety of foods in one week, often over 100 different ingredients! Eating a wide range of fruits and vegetables ensures that you're getting a diverse array of vitamins, minerals, and fibre. For example, sweet potatoes (satsumaimo) are a popular snack in Japan, and they're full of fibre and antioxidants, perfect for digestion and immune support. Japanese people also love their fermented vegetables, such as tsukemono (pickled vegetables), which are excellent for gut health and digestion. And let's not forget about the miso soup, a staple in Japanese meals, often made with seaweed, tofu, and seasonal vegetables perfect for warming the body and nourishing the soul.

3. **Opt for Organic Produce and Low-Chemical Farming**

While the Japanese diet is primarily focused on fresh, whole foods, there is also a strong emphasis on organic and naturally grown produce. Organic farming, known as yukiguni in Japan, is growing in popularity due to its focus on low-chemical and sustainable practices. Japanese consumers often prefer seasonal, locally sourced, and organically grown vegetables. Koshihikari rice, considered one of the finest types of Japanese rice, is often grown with care and attention to the environment. When possible, try to buy organic produce, especially in your local Japanese market, where you can find shojin ryori (Buddhist temple cuisine) ingredients, which focus on plant-based and organic food.

4. **Consume Fish and Fish Oils**

The Japanese are known for their high consumption of fish, which plays a central role in their diet. Sushi and sashimi, with their delicate cuts of raw fish, are iconic examples of Japanese cuisine that promote healthy omega-3 fatty acids. Fish such as salmon, mackerel, and tuna are staples in the Japanese diet and are rich in essential fatty acids that support brain health, reduce inflammation, and boost heart health. Even in traditional Japanese breakfast sets, you'll find grilled salmon or sardines served alongside rice and miso soup. These fish oils also provide essential nucleic acids for cell repair, and omega-3 fatty acids are key in reducing the risk of chronic diseases. If you don't eat fish, consider supplementing your diet with seaweed, seeds, or nuts, all of which contain plant-based omega-3s.

5. **Cut Down on Dairy**

Dairy is not a significant part of the traditional Japanese diet, and it's something many people in Japan naturally avoid. While dairy products like cheese and milk are consumed in small quantities, they are not as central to meals as they are in Western cultures. In fact, most Japanese people have adapted to lactose intolerance. Instead, they opt for plant-based alternatives like soymilk (which is a great source of calcium) and tofu, which is made from soybeans. Soy-based foods, such as edamame and miso, offer plenty of protein and essential nutrients without the heavy fat content of dairy. The Japanese also prefer to get their calcium from green leafy vegetables such as spinach (horenso), shiso leaves, and seaweed (kombu), all of which are rich in calcium and other minerals.

6. **Cut Down on Sugar and Saturated Fats**

The Japanese diet is naturally low in added sugars and saturated fats, focusing instead on wholesome, unprocessed foods. You won't find sugary snacks or heavily processed desserts commonly consumed in Japan. Instead, Japanese sweets, known as wagashi, are often made with ingredients like adzuki beans, mochi, and matcha, which provide a naturally sweet flavour without the need for refined sugars. Mochi, a chewy rice cake, is a popular treat, often served with a small amount of sweet red bean paste. The Japanese also use healthy fats in their cooking, such as sesame oil, olive oil, and fish oils, rather than heavily processed vegetable oils that can lead to inflammation and weight gain. Keep your fats healthy by incorporating avocados, olive oil, and nuts into your meals, and enjoy the naturally sweet taste of Japanese desserts without the added sugar.

7. **Avoid Food Additives**

Japanese food culture places a high value on the purity and simplicity of ingredients, with minimal use of artificial additives, preservatives, or flavour enhancers. Umami, the fifth taste, is cherished in Japan and can be found in natural sources like miso, soy sauce, and dashi (fish broth). Japanese people use these flavourful, natural ingredients to bring depth to their food without relying on artificial flavourings. The Japanese also pay close attention to food packaging, and you'll often find products with fewer preservatives. As you move away from processed foods, try to focus on whole, minimally processed ingredients and experiment with making your own sauces and seasonings.

8. **Strive for an Alkalizing Diet**

In Japan, the emphasis is on a balanced diet, which includes a variety of alkalizing foods. The Japanese diet is naturally low in acid-forming foods like meat and dairy, and instead, it's rich in alkalizing vegetables, such as daikon, spinach, kale, sweet potatoes, and seaweed. To maintain balance, aim for a diet filled with fresh fruits and vegetables, especially those that are green and leafy, to help keep your pH levels in balance and reduce the risk of chronic disease.

9. **Eat Smaller Portions and Mindfully**

One of the most profound aspects of the Japanese approach to food is their attitude toward portion sizes. Kaiseki meals, which are multi-course meals served in traditional tea houses, are presented in small portions with carefully considered flavours. Even in a simple Japanese home, meals are served in a variety of small bowls, allowing the diner to savour each dish slowly. Eating in this way not only aids digestion but also allows for mindfulness and appreciation of the meal. The Japanese principle of 'Hara Hachi Bu', which means "eat until you are 80% full," encourages you to listen to your body and stop eating before you feel stuffed. This practice helps with weight management and overall health.

10. **Supplement with Traditional Herbal Remedies**
In Japan, herbal medicine plays an important role in supporting health. Kampo, the Japanese form of traditional Chinese medicine, includes a variety of herbs that support digestion, boost immunity, and improve energy levels. Some of the most popular herbs in Japan include ginseng, ginger, and matcha, which is loaded with antioxidants and promotes detoxification. Herbal teas, like sencha (green tea), hojicha (roasted green tea), and genmaicha (green tea with roasted brown rice), are common in Japanese homes and provide a calming, antioxidant-rich beverage.

By adopting some of these principles into your daily routine, you'll not only nourish your body but also cultivate the mindfulness, appreciation, and balance that are central to Japanese food culture. The Japanese way of eating isn't just about food, it's about celebrating life, connecting with nature, and honouring the traditions passed down through generations. So, take a moment to savour each bite, enjoy the beauty of your meal, and nourish your body with the wholesome, delicious food of Japan.

The Japanese diet is often linked to longevity and overall health, and there's a wealth of scientific research supporting this connection. Here are some key aspects of the Japanese diet that contribute to its health benefits:

1. **Rich in Nutrient-Dense Foods:** The Japanese diet is abundant in vegetables, fruits, seaweed, and fish, all of which are packed with essential nutrients, vitamins, and minerals. These foods provide antioxidants and anti-inflammatory compounds that protect against chronic diseases.

2. **High in Omega-3 Fatty Acids:** Fish, a staple in the Japanese diet, is rich in omega-3 fatty acids, which are known to support heart health, reduce inflammation, and improve brain function. Regular fish consumption is linked to a lower risk of heart disease and stroke.

3. **Low in Saturated Fats:** The Japanese diet is typically low in red meat and saturated fats, which helps maintain healthy cholesterol levels and reduces the risk of cardiovascular diseases.

4. **Balanced Portions and Variety:** Japanese meals often consist of small, balanced portions with a variety of foods. This approach not only prevents overeating but also ensures a diverse intake of nutrients.

5. **Fermented Foods:** Fermented foods like miso, natto, and pickled vegetables are common in the Japanese diet. These foods are rich in probiotics, which promote gut health, enhance digestion, and boost the immune system.

6. **Green Tea Consumption:** Regular consumption of green tea, which is high in antioxidants, is associated

with reduced risk of heart disease and certain cancers, as well as improved brain health.

7. **Mindful Eating Practices:** The Japanese culture emphasizes mindful eating, savouring each bite, and appreciating the food's flavours and textures. This practice can lead to better digestion and a more satisfying eating experience.

8. **Low Sugar and Processed Foods:** The traditional Japanese diet is low in sugar and processed foods, reducing the risk of obesity, diabetes, and other metabolic disorders.

Overall, the Japanese diet's emphasis on fresh, whole foods, balanced nutrition, and mindful eating practices contributes significantly to longevity and a lower incidence of chronic diseases.

I hope this exploration has inspired you to embark on a journey of journaling about meal planning, healthy eating, and nourishing your body for longevity. By documenting your thoughts and plans, you can create a personalized roadmap to better health and well-being.

Start by reflecting on your current eating habits and identifying areas for improvement. Consider incorporating more nutrient-dense foods, such as fresh vegetables, fruits, whole grains, and lean proteins, into your meals. Explore the benefits of the traditional Japanese diet, which emphasize balance, variety, and mindful eating.

Use your journal to set realistic goals for meal planning, whether it's preparing meals in advance, experimenting with new recipes, or trying out different cuisines that prioritize health. Track your progress and celebrate small victories along the way, noting how these changes impact your energy levels, mood, and overall health.

As you journal, consider the broader impact of your dietary choices on longevity. Reflect on how nourishing your body with wholesome foods can enhance your quality of life, support your physical and mental well-being, and contribute to a longer, healthier life.

Let your journal be a source of inspiration and motivation, guiding you towards a lifestyle that prioritizes health, vitality, and longevity.

ACTION - Go to the journal prompts at the end of this recipe section, start meal planning and start looking at these amazingly delicious, easy to cook, recipes below.

1. **Miso Soup (味噌汁 / Miso Shiru)**
Prep + Cook Time: 10–15 minutes

Serves: 2–3

Ingredients:

- 3 cups (750 ml) water
- 1½ tablespoons miso paste (white or red, depending on your taste)
- 1 teaspoon dashi granules (or use kombu/shiitake stock if vegan)
- ½ cup silken tofu, cubed
- 1 sheet of nori (seaweed), cut into small strips or squares
- 1–2 tablespoons chopped green onions (scallions)
- Optional: a few slices of shiitake mushrooms, wakame seaweed, or baby spinach

Instructions:

1. **Prepare the broth**
    In a saucepan, bring the water to a gentle simmer. Add the dashi granules and stir until dissolved (or use your prepared kombu/shiitake stock if going plant-based).
2. **Add extras**
    If you're using mushrooms or wakame, add them now and let them cook for 2–3 minutes until tender.
3. **Add tofu and nori**
    Gently slide in the cubed tofu and nori pieces. Simmer for another 1–2 minutes to warm through.

4. **Stir in the miso (important step!)**
   Turn off the heat. In a small bowl, scoop a bit of the hot broth and dissolve the miso paste into it, then stir this mixture back into the pot. Never boil miso, it kills the beneficial enzymes and probiotics!
5. **Garnish and serve**
   Sprinkle chopped green onions over the top. Serve immediately in small bowls and enjoy mindfully.

Wellness Tip:

Miso is rich in probiotics, antioxidants, and B vitamins. Combining it with tofu and seaweed offers gut-friendly, mineral-rich nourishment—perfect for digestion and longevity, the Japanese way.

Mindfulness Tip for Making Miso Soup

As you prepare miso soup, take a moment to slow down and engage your senses fully. Listen to the gentle simmer of the dashi, notice the earthy aroma of the miso as it dissolves, and feel the warmth of the steam rising from the pot. Stir slowly and with intention, treating each movement as an act of care.

Let the simplicity of the ingredients remind you: wellness begins with presence. Just like miso soup (humble, nourishing, and grounding), your small, mindful actions can bring warmth and balance to your day.

Itadakimasu. Let this dish nourish not just your body, but your spirit.

"Gochisōsama deshita" after eating (Thank you for the meal).

2. Chicken Teriyaki (照り焼きチキン / Teriyaki Chicken)
Prep + Cook Time: 25 minutes

Serves: 2–3

Ingredients:

- 2 boneless, skinless chicken thighs (or breasts if preferred)
- 1 tablespoon neutral oil (like avocado or light olive oil)
- 1 tablespoon cornstarch (optional, for crispier texture)

For the Teriyaki Sauce:

- 3 tablespoons low-sodium soy sauce
- 2 tablespoons mirin (or a mix of rice vinegar + a pinch of sugar)
- 1 tablespoon honey or maple syrup
- 1 tablespoon sake (optional for authenticity; can substitute water)
- 1 teaspoon grated ginger (fresh is best!)
- 1 small garlic clove, minced

Instructions:

1. **Prep the chicken**
   Pat the chicken dry and (optional) lightly dust with cornstarch for a nice crisp sear. This step helps create a slightly caramelized surface.
2. **Make the sauce**
   In a small bowl, whisk together soy sauce, mirin, honey, sake, ginger, and garlic. Set aside.

3. **Cook the chicken**
Heat oil in a non-stick pan over medium heat. Add the chicken and cook 4–5 minutes on each side, or until golden and cooked through.
4. **Add the sauce**
Reduce heat slightly. Pour the teriyaki sauce over the chicken. Let it bubble gently for 2–3 minutes, turning the chicken so it's well coated and glazed.
5. **Slice and serve**
Remove chicken, slice into strips, and drizzle with remaining sauce from the pan. Serve with steamed rice and a side of sautéed greens or pickled veggies.

Wellness Tip:

Using low-sodium soy sauce and natural sweeteners like **honey** helps reduce refined sugar and salt intake while still delivering bold flavour. Pairing this dish with **brown rice and fibre-rich vegetables** helps balance blood sugar, support digestion, and extend satiety—perfect principles from the Japanese approach to nourishment.

Mindfulness Tip for Making Chicken Teriyaki

As you prepare your chicken teriyaki, be fully present with each step—slicing the chicken with care, watching the sauce bubble and caramelize, and noticing the rich, savory aroma filling your kitchen. Instead of rushing, treat the cooking process as a peaceful ritual.

Allow the transformation of simple ingredients into a delicious dish to remind you of your own capacity for change and growth. Let each stir, each glaze, be a moment of gratitude—for the nourishment you're creating and the time you're gifting yourself. Cooking can be more than a task; it can be a moment of grounding and calm in your day.

Itadakimasu. Let this dish nourish not just your body, but your spirit.

"Gochisōsama deshita" after eating (Thank you for the meal).

3. Vegetable Tempura (野菜の天ぷら / Yasai no Tempura)
Prep + Cook Time: 30 minutes

Serves: 2–3

Ingredients:

Vegetables (choose 4–5 of your favourites):

- Sweet potato (peeled and sliced into thin rounds)
- Carrot (cut into thin sticks)
- Zucchini (sliced into rounds or strips)
- Bell pepper (cut into strips)
- Broccoli or green beans
- Shiitake or enoki mushrooms

Tip: Keep the cuts thin so they cook quickly in the oil.

Batter:

- ½ cup all-purpose flour (or rice flour for extra lightness)
- ½ cup ice-cold sparkling water (or just cold water)
- 1 tablespoon cornstarch or potato starch
- 1 egg (optional, for richer texture)
- Pinch of salt

Oil for frying:

- Neutral oil like sunflower, canola, or avocado (for deep frying)

Dipping Sauce:

- ¼ cup soy sauce
- 2 tablespoons mirin or rice vinegar
- 1 tablespoon grated daikon (optional)
- A dash of grated ginger (optional)

Instructions:

1. **Prep the vegetables**
   Wash and slice vegetables uniformly. Pat them dry completely to avoid oil splatter.
2. **Make the dipping sauce**
   Mix soy sauce, mirin, daikon, and ginger in a small bowl. Set aside.
3. **Prepare the batter**
   In a bowl, gently whisk flour, starch, and a pinch of salt. Add cold water (and egg, if using). Don't overmix—the batter should be slightly lumpy. Cold batter is key to crispy tempura!
4. **Heat the oil**
   In a deep pan, heat 1½–2 inches of oil to 170–180°C (340–360°F). Test with a small drop of batter—it should sizzle and rise quickly.
5. **Fry the vegetables**
   Dip each vegetable into the batter, then carefully place in the hot oil. Don't overcrowd the pan. Fry until lightly golden and crispy (about 2–3 minutes per batch). Remove and drain on paper towels.
6. **Serve immediately**

Serve hot with dipping sauce and a bowl of rice or miso soup.

Wellness Tip:

While tempura is a fried dish, it can still be part of a balanced Japanese-style meal when paired with steamed rice, miso soup, and a fresh salad. Using a light batter, seasonal vegetables, and quality oil keeps it nourishing. And eating it slowly, with gratitude as in Japanese mealtime customs helps prevent overeating and enhances digestion.

Mindfulness Tip for Making Vegetable Tempura

When making vegetable tempura, let the process become a meditative practice. As you slice each vegetable, observe its colours, textures, and natural patterns, each piece unique and beautiful in its simplicity.

When dipping into the batter and placing it gently in the hot oil, listen to the soft sizzle. Stay present. Don't rush. Be aware of your breath as you move with care and precision.

This is more than just cooking, it's an invitation to slow down and honour the moment. Like in traditional Japanese culture, finding beauty in the ordinary brings peace to the mind and joy to the heart. Let the act of cooking connect you back to the here and now.

Itadakimasu. Let this dish nourish not just your body, but your spirit.

"Gochisōsama deshita" after eating (Thank you for the meal).

Air Fryer Vegetable Tempura Instructions

Prep + Cook Time: 30–35 minutes

Serves: 2–3

Ingredients

(Same as original recipe, with slight adjustments)

Vegetables:

- Choose 4–5: sweet potato, carrot, zucchini, bell pepper, green beans, mushrooms, etc.
- Slice thinly for faster cooking.

Light Batter:

- ½ cup all-purpose flour (or rice flour)
- ½ cup ice-cold sparkling water
- 1 tablespoon cornstarch or potato starch
- 1 egg (optional)
- Pinch of salt
- 1–2 tablespoons neutral oil (like avocado or grapeseed, for brushing/spraying)

Optional: Panko breadcrumbs for extra crunch (lightly pressed onto veggies)

Instructions

1. **Prep vegetables**
   Wash, dry, and cut your vegetables thinly and uniformly.
2. **Preheat your air fryer**
   Set it to **200°C / 390°F** for 3–5 minutes.
3. **Make the batter**
   Whisk flour, cornstarch, salt, and cold water (plus egg if using) until just combined. Keep it cold and slightly lumpy for best results.
4. **Coat the vegetables**
   Dip each piece into the batter. Shake off the excess. Optional: press gently into panko for added texture.
5. **Light oil spray or brush**
   Lightly spray or brush both sides of each battered vegetable with oil. This helps crisping in the air fryer.
6. **Air fry in batches**
   Place vegetables in a single layer in the air fryer basket. Do not overcrowd.
   Air fry for 7–10 minutes, flipping halfway through and lightly respraying if needed.
   Cook until golden and crisp.
7. **Serve immediately**
   Best enjoyed hot, with your dipping sauce (soy sauce + mirin + ginger).

Wellness Tip:

Air-frying significantly reduces oil use while keeping the tempura light and crispy. Paired with miso soup or a seaweed salad, this becomes a nutrient-rich, heart-friendly version of a traditional favourite. Eating mindfully and seasonally, just like in Japanese food culture, enhances the wellness benefits.

Mindfulness Tip for Making Vegetable Tempura

When making vegetable tempura, let the process become a meditative practice. As you slice each vegetable, observe its colours, textures, and natural patterns, each piece unique and beautiful in its simplicity.

When dipping into the batter and placing it gently in the hot oil, listen to the soft sizzle. Stay present. Don't rush. Be aware of your breath as you move with care and precision.

This is more than just cooking, it's an invitation to slow down and honour the moment. Like in traditional Japanese culture, finding beauty in the ordinary brings peace to the mind and joy to the heart. Let the act of cooking connect you back to the here and now.

Itadakimasu. Let this dish nourish not just your body, but your spirit.

"Gochisōsama deshita" after eating (Thank you for the meal).

4. Salmon Onigiri (鮭おにぎり / Rice Balls with Salmon) (and options)

Prep & Cook Time: 35–40 minutes

Serves: 4–6 onigiri

Ingredients

For the Rice:

- 2 cups Japanese short-grain rice (sushi rice)
- 2½ cups water
- Pinch of salt
- Optional: 1 tbsp rice vinegar for extra flavour

For the Filling:

- 1 salmon fillet (about 120–150g), cooked and flaked
- ½ tsp soy sauce
- ½ tsp sesame oil
- Optional: sprinkle of toasted sesame seeds

Other Filling Options:

- **Tuna mayo:** canned tuna + Japanese mayo + soy sauce
- **Umeboshi:** pickled plum (traditional and tart)
- **Avocado + sesame:** mashed avocado + toasted sesame
- **Kimchi:** finely chopped for a spicy kick
- **Miso eggplant:** sautéed eggplant cubes with miso glaze

285

To Shape:

- Nori (seaweed) sheets, cut into strips or squares
- Bowl of water + pinch of salt (for wetting your hands)

Instructions

1. **Cook the rice**
   Rinse rice until water runs clear. Cook in a rice cooker or pot with water. Let it steam for 10 mins after cooking.
2. **Prepare the salmon filling**
   Pan-fry or bake the salmon, season with soy sauce and sesame oil, then flake with a fork. Let cool.
3. **Shape the onigiri**
   - Wet your hands with salted water (this keeps the rice from sticking and adds flavour).
   - Scoop about ½ cup of warm rice into your palm, flatten it slightly.
   - Place 1 tbsp of salmon in the centre.
   - Gently fold the rice around the filling, then shape into a triangle or oval.
4. **Wrap with nori**
   Press a strip or small square of nori on one side for easy handling.
5. **Serve or store**
   Eat immediately or wrap in cling film and store in the fridge (best eaten within 24 hours).

Wellness Tip

Onigiri is a beautifully balanced snack, rich in complex carbs, customizable protein, and naturally low in additives. By using fillings like salmon (high in omega-3s), avocado (good fats), or miso eggplant (fermented foods), you nourish your body with anti-inflammatory, gut-friendly, and brain-boosting nutrients.

Eating onigiri mindfully, perhaps with a cup of green tea, which can turn a simple meal into a calming, nourishing ritual.

Mindfulness Tip for Making Onigiri

As you prepare onigiri, treat each step as a quiet ritual. Feel the warmth and texture of the rice in your hands, soft, nourishing, and grounding. Shape each rice ball slowly and intentionally, noticing how the grains come together with gentle pressure.

Focus on your breath as you add your chosen filling—whether it's comforting salmon, tangy umeboshi, or savoury miso, acknowledging the care that goes into nourishing yourself or a loved one.

Let this moment remind you: like onigiri, life is made of simple, meaningful gestures. Be present, be gentle, and infuse your food with calm intention.

Itadakimasu. Let this dish nourish not just your body, but your spirit.

"Gochisōsama deshita" after eating (Thank you for the meal).

5. Chirashi Sushi (ちらし寿司 / Scattered Sushi Bowl), A vibrant, wellness-packed sushi bowl

Prep & Cook Time: 40 minutes

Serves: 2–3

Ingredients

For the Sushi Rice:

- 2 cups Japanese short-grain rice
- 2½ cups water
- 3 tbsp rice vinegar
- 1½ tbsp sugar
- ½ tsp salt

Toppings (choose a variety):

- 100g sashimi-grade salmon or tuna, sliced or cubed
- 1 egg, beaten and cooked into a thin omelette, then sliced into strips
- ½ avocado, sliced
- ½ cucumber, julienned
- Cooked and seasoned shiitake mushrooms or edamame
- Pickled ginger (gari)
- Toasted sesame seeds
- Nori (seaweed) strips or flakes
- Optional: tobiko (fish roe), radish sprouts, or microgreens

Instructions

1. **Prepare the rice**
   Rinse the rice until water runs clear. Cook in rice cooker or pot with 2½ cups of water. Let it steam for 10 minutes after cooking.
2. **Make the sushi vinegar**
   In a small bowl, mix rice vinegar, sugar, and salt until dissolved. Gently fold into the cooked rice using a wooden spoon. Let cool slightly.
3. **Prepare your toppings**
   While the rice cools, prepare all toppings. Cook and season shiitake if using, slice veggies and fish, and prepare omelette strips.
4. **Assemble the Chirashi Sushi**
   Spoon the sushi rice into a bowl or platter. Artfully scatter your toppings across the surface, aiming for a colourful, balanced look. Garnish with sesame seeds and nori strips.

Wellness Tip

Chirashi sushi is not only beautiful, but it also supports **balanced nutrition**. With complex carbs from rice, protein from fish or tofu, and antioxidant-rich veggies, it's a complete meal. The act of arranging the dish can also be **meditative**, encouraging mindfulness and joy in food preparation.

Wellness boost: Add **fermented toppings** like pickled ginger or seasoned mushrooms for gut health, and **omega-3 rich fish** for brain and heart support.

Mindfulness Tip When Making Chirashi Sushi

As you prepare chirashi sushi, approach it like an art form, each ingredient a brushstroke, each colour a celebration of nature's palette.

Take a moment to connect with the freshness of each topping, feel the textures, notice the vibrant hues of vegetables, fish, or egg. As you gently place each element atop the seasoned rice, breathe deeply and move slowly, letting the arrangement unfold with care rather than haste.

Chirashi sushi invites balance, not only in flavour, but in mindset. Let it remind you to find beauty in variety, harmony in contrast, and joy in mindful creation. This bowl is more than food; it's a reflection of presence and appreciation.

Itadakimasu. Let this dish nourish not just your body, but your spirit.

"Gochisōsama deshita" after eating (Thank you for the meal).

6. Beef Gyudon (牛丼 / Beef Bowl), A savoury, satisfying one-bowl meal

Prep & Cook Time: 25 minutes

Serves: 2

Ingredients

- 250g thinly sliced beef (ribeye or sirloin works best)
- 1 medium onion, thinly sliced
- 1 cup dashi stock (or use water + 1 tsp dashi powder)
- 3 tbsp soy sauce
- 2 tbsp mirin
- 1 tbsp sake (optional)
- 1 tbsp sugar (adjust to taste)
- 2 bowls cooked Japanese rice
- Optional toppings:
  - Pickled ginger (beni shoga)
  - Soft boiled egg or onsen tamago
  - Chopped spring onions
  - Shichimi togarashi (Japanese chili blend)

Instructions

1. **Prepare the sauce**
   In a medium saucepan, combine dashi, soy sauce, mirin, sake, and sugar. Bring to a gentle simmer over medium heat.
2. **Cook the onion**
   Add the sliced onion and cook until softened, about 5 minutes.

3. **Add the beef**

   Add the thinly sliced beef to the pot, separating the slices as you place them in. Simmer gently until the beef is just cooked through (about 3–4 minutes).

4. **Assemble the bowls**

   Divide the cooked rice into two bowls. Spoon the beef and onion mixture on top, then drizzle some of the sauce over the rice.

5. **Garnish**

   Add your preferred toppings—such as pickled ginger, soft egg, or scallions.

Wellness Tip

Beef Gyudon can be a great high-protein, iron-rich meal, especially when made with lean cuts and served with vegetables or fermented pickles. To balance the glycemic load, use brown rice or mix white rice with barley (mugi gohan), a popular Japanese addition that boosts fibre and improves digestion.

Mindful Eating Tip: Enjoy Gyudon slowly, with gratitude—following the spirit of *Ichiju Sansai* (one soup, three sides) to create a well-rounded, satisfying meal.

Itadakimasu. Let this dish nourish not just your body, but your spirit.

"Gochisōsama deshita" after eating (Thank you for the meal).

7. Tamago Yaki (卵焼き / Japanese Rolled Omelette)
Prep & Cook Time: 15 minutes

Serves: 2

Ingredients

- 3 large eggs
- 1 tbsp mirin
- 1 tsp soy sauce (or tamari for gluten-free)
- 1 tsp sugar (optional for sweetness)
- Pinch of salt
- Oil for cooking (e.g., sesame or neutral oil)

Instructions

1. **Prepare the egg mixture**
   In a mixing bowl, gently beat the eggs with mirin, soy sauce, sugar (if using), and a pinch of salt. Try not to over-beat, just mix until well combined.
2. **Heat your pan**
   Use a small non-stick frying pan or a rectangular tamagoyaki pan if you have one. Lightly oil the pan and heat over medium-low.
3. **Cook in layers**
   - Pour a thin layer of the egg mixture into the pan.
   - Let it set slightly, then gently roll it toward one side of the pan.
   - Re-oil the exposed pan and pour in another thin layer, lifting the cooked roll to let egg flow underneath.

- Once it sets, roll again. Repeat until all the egg is used.

4. **Shape and slice**
Once done, let the roll rest for a minute, then slice into even pieces.

5. **Serve warm or chilled**
Serve with rice, in a bento box, or as a protein-packed snack.

Wellness Tip

Tamagoyaki is a wonderful source of high-quality protein and B vitamins, which are essential for energy and brain function. Adding a bit of dashi stock to the mix (for an authentic version) boosts the umami flavour and adds trace minerals that support nerve and muscle health.

Mindfulness Tip: Making Tamagoyaki requires patience, rhythm, and presence, making it a perfect opportunity to practice *Kanso* (simplicity) and *Shokunin* (craftsmanship) in the kitchen.

Itadakimasu. Let this dish nourish not just your body, but your spirit.

"Gochisōsama deshita" after eating (Thank you for the meal).

8. Yakisoba (焼きそば / Stir-Fried Noodles)
Prep & Cook Time: 20 minutes

Serves: 2-3

Ingredients

- 200g (7 oz) yakisoba noodles (or any thin fresh noodles like ramen or soba)
- 1 tbsp sesame oil (or vegetable oil)
- 1 small onion, thinly sliced
- 1/2 bell pepper, thinly sliced
- 1 medium carrot, julienned or thinly sliced
- 1/2 cup cabbage, shredded (or other greens like spinach or bok choy)
- 2-3 tbsp soy sauce (or tamari for gluten-free)
- 1 tbsp oyster sauce (optional for umami flavour)
- 1 tsp mirin (optional for a touch of sweetness)
- 1 tsp Worcestershire sauce (optional for deeper flavour)
- 1 tbsp rice vinegar (optional for a light tang)
- 1/2 tsp grated ginger (optional for an aromatic kick)
- A sprinkle of sesame seeds and chopped green onions for garnish

Instructions

1. **Prepare the noodles**
   If using fresh yakisoba noodles, simply loosen them in boiling water for 2-3 minutes and drain. If using pre-cooked, follow the instructions on the package. Set aside.

2. **Sauté the veggies**

   Heat the sesame oil in a large frying pan or wok over medium heat. Add the onions and sauté until softened (about 2-3 minutes). Add the bell pepper, carrot, and cabbage, and stir-fry for another 3-4 minutes until the vegetables are tender but still slightly crisp.

3. **Stir-fry the noodles**

   Push the veggies to one side of the pan, then add the noodles to the empty side of the pan. Stir-fry for 2-3 minutes until the noodles are heated through and lightly browned.

4. **Flavour it up**

   Drizzle soy sauce, oyster sauce, mirin, Worcestershire sauce, and rice vinegar over the noodles and veggies. Add the grated ginger, if using. Toss everything together until well coated and evenly combined. Stir-fry for another minute or so, letting the flavours meld together.

5. **Serve and garnish**

   Divide the yakisoba between plates, sprinkle with sesame seeds and chopped green onions. Serve hot and enjoy!

Wellness Tip

Yakisoba is a perfect balanced meal, offering fibre and vitamins from the vegetables (carrots, bell peppers, cabbage), and complex carbs from the noodles. The inclusion of sesame oil provides heart-healthy fats, and the use of soy sauce adds a good amount of umami without being overly salty when used in moderation. For extra protein, you can add tofu, chicken, or shrimp.

Mindful Eating Tip: While eating your yakisoba, take a moment to appreciate the harmony of flavours—sweet, savoury, tangy, and umami. Practice mindfulness by savouring each bite slowly, fully experiencing the textures and aromas. This helps you become more present, reduces overeating, and enhances digestion.

Itadakimasu. Let this dish nourish not just your body, but your spirit.

"Gochisōsama deshita" after eating (Thank you for the meal).

9. **Okonomiyaki (お好み焼き / Savory Japanese Pancake)**

Okonomiyaki is a savoury, pancake-like dish from Japan that's often packed with vegetables, proteins, and topped with a delicious sauce. It's versatile and can be made to suit your tastes, and today we're making it simple, healthy, and with a gluten-free option!

Prep & Cook Time: 20-25 minutes

Serves: 2-3

Ingredients

For the Pancake Batter:

- 1 cup all-purpose flour (or gluten-free flour blend)
- 1/4 cup cornstarch (for extra crispiness)
- 1/2 tsp baking powder
- 1/2 cup water (or dashi stock for more depth of flavour)
- 1 large egg
- 1 tbsp soy sauce (or tamari for gluten-free)
- 1 tsp sesame oil

For the Filling:

- 1/2 small cabbage, shredded
- 1 small carrot, grated
- 1/4 cup green onions, chopped
- 1/2 cup cooked chicken (or shrimp, tofu, or pork) — optional
- 1/2 cup cooked bacon or ham — optional

For the Topping (optional):

- Okonomiyaki sauce (or substitute with a mixture of Worcestershire sauce, soy sauce, and a little honey)
- A drizzle of mayonnaise (preferably Japanese Kewpie mayonnaise for a creamy texture)
- Bonito flakes (dried fish flakes)
- A sprinkle of seaweed flakes (nori)

Instructions

1. **Prepare the batter**
   In a large mixing bowl, combine the flour, cornstarch, and baking powder. Add the water (or dashi stock) and whisk until smooth. Beat in the egg, soy sauce, and sesame oil until well incorporated.

2. **Prepare the filling**
   Add the shredded cabbage, grated carrot, and chopped green onions to the batter. If you're adding any protein (chicken, shrimp, bacon, or tofu), mix those in as well. Stir everything together until evenly combined.

3. **Cook the okonomiyaki**
   Heat a non-stick pan or griddle over medium heat and brush with a bit of sesame oil. Pour the okonomiyaki batter into the pan, shaping it into a round pancake, about 1-inch thick. Cook for 3-4 minutes, until the edges start to firm up and the bottom is golden brown. Flip carefully using a spatula and cook for another 3-4 minutes on the other side, until golden brown and cooked through.

4. **Serve and top**
   Once cooked, transfer to a plate. Drizzle with okonomiyaki sauce (or your Worcestershire-honey mixture), a bit of mayonnaise, and top with bonito flakes and seaweed flakes.

Wellness Tip

Okonomiyaki is a well-rounded dish offering fibre from the cabbage and carrots, protein from the meat or tofu, and healthy fats from sesame oil. The dish also contains a variety of antioxidants from the veggies and the optional seaweed flakes. You can make it even healthier by opting for gluten-free flour, reducing sodium with a low-sodium soy sauce, and adding more vegetables for extra nutrition. It's a great meal to support digestion and metabolism, especially when eaten as part of a balanced diet.

Mindfulness Tip: While eating your okonomiyaki, try the practice of mindful eating. Before you take the first bite, pause and appreciate the colours, textures, and aroma of the food. Take small, thoughtful bites and chew slowly. This practice enhances digestion and helps you feel more connected to the meal, appreciating the ingredients and the nourishment they provide to your body.

Okonomiyaki is not only delicious and nutritious but also embodies the Japanese principle of wabi-sabi, finding beauty in imperfection. Whether you choose the classic ingredients or make it your own, each bite is a reminder of the joy of simplicity and mindfulness. Enjoy!

Itadakimasu. Let this dish nourish not just your body, but your spirit.

"Gochisōsama deshita" after eating (Thank you for the meal).

10. Nasu Dengaku (茄子田楽 / Miso-Glazed Eggplant)

A simple, elegant Japanese side dish bursting with umami flavour.

Prep & Cook Time: 25 minutes

Serves: 2

Ingredients

- 2 small Japanese eggplants (or 1 large globe eggplant)
- 1 tbsp sesame oil (or neutral oil like avocado oil)
- Toasted sesame seeds and sliced spring onions for garnish (optional)

For the Miso Glaze (Dengaku Miso):

- 2 tbsp miso paste (white or red; white is milder and slightly sweeter)
- 1 tbsp mirin
- 1 tbsp sake (or water if avoiding alcohol)
- 1 tsp sugar (or maple syrup for a natural alternative)
- 1 tsp rice vinegar (optional, for brightness)

Instructions

1. **Prepare the eggplant**
   Cut the eggplants in half lengthwise. Score the flesh with a crisscross pattern (be careful not to cut through the skin). This helps the glaze penetrate and cook evenly.

2. **Roast or pan-fry the eggplant**

Brush the cut side with sesame oil. You can either:

o **Roast**: Place cut side up on a baking sheet and roast at 200°C (400°F) for about 15–20 minutes until soft and lightly browned.

o **Pan-fry**: Heat a pan over medium heat and cook cut side down until golden brown and tender, about 4–5 minutes per side.

3. **Make the glaze**

While the eggplant cooks, whisk together the miso paste, mirin, sake (or water), sugar, and rice vinegar in a small saucepan over low heat. Stir until smooth and slightly thickened (2–3 minutes). Remove from heat.

4. **Glaze and broil (optional)**

Once the eggplant is cooked, spoon the miso glaze generously over the cut surface. If you'd like a caramelized finish, place the glazed eggplant under a broiler for 2–3 minutes.

5. **Serve**

Garnish with toasted sesame seeds and finely sliced spring onions. Serve hot or warm as a side dish or part of a Japanese-style meal.

Wellness Tip

Eggplant is high in fibre, low in calories, and packed with antioxidants like nasunin (found in the purple skin), which supports brain and cellular health. The miso provides beneficial probiotics and enzymes that support gut health and immune function, especially when it's fermented naturally.

Mindfulness Tip

When preparing and eating nasu dengaku, use it as a moment to practice presence and gratitude. Notice the vibrant purple of the eggplant, the rich aroma of the miso, and the sizzling sound as it cooks. Eat slowly, savouring the balance of sweet, salty, and umami flavours, and appreciate the nourishment and care put into a humble vegetable turned into a beautiful dish.

Nasu Dengaku is a reminder that simple ingredients, when treated with attention and care, can become deeply satisfying and nourishing, a perfect example of Japanese food philosophy in action.

Itadakimasu. Let this dish nourish not just your body, but your spirit.

"Gochisōsama deshita" after eating (Thank you for the meal).

11. Kitsune Udon (きつねうどん / Udon Noodles with Fried Tofu)

Prep time: 15 minutes

Serves 2

Ingredients:

- 2 portions udon noodles (fresh or frozen)
- 2 pieces aburaage (fried tofu pouches)
- 2 ½ cups dashi broth (instant dashi powder or homemade)
- 2 tbsp soy sauce
- 1 tbsp mirin
- 1 tsp sugar (optional)
- 1 tbsp sake (optional)
- 2 spring onions, finely sliced
- Optional toppings: shichimi togarashi (7-spice mix), wakame seaweed, narutomaki (fish cake)

Instructions:

1. **Prepare the Aburaage:**
   o Pour boiling water over the aburaage to remove excess oil.
   o Gently squeeze out the water and slice each piece in half.
   o In a small saucepan, combine ½ cup water, 1 tbsp soy sauce, 1 tbsp mirin, and 1 tsp sugar. Add aburaage and simmer for 5–6 minutes until it absorbs the flavour. Set aside.

2. **Make the Broth:**
   - ○ In a pot, heat 2 cups of dashi broth.
   - ○ Add 1 tbsp soy sauce, 1 tbsp mirin, and 1 tbsp sake (if using).
   - ○ Taste and adjust seasoning (add a pinch of salt or a dash more soy sauce if needed).
3. **Cook the Udon:**
   - ○ Boil udon noodles according to package instructions. Drain and rinse briefly under warm water.
4. **Assemble the Bowls:**
   - ○ Divide noodles into bowls.
   - ○ Pour the hot broth over the noodles.
   - ○ Top each bowl with 1 piece of sweet aburaage.
   - ○ Garnish with chopped spring onions and optional toppings.

Wellness Tip:

Udon is a gentle, nourishing food that is easy on digestion and perfect for calming the body. The plant-based protein from tofu is also a heart-healthy alternative to meat. Choose low-sodium soy sauce to keep the dish light and supportive of blood pressure balance.

Mindfulness Tip:

As you assemble your bowl, let it be a meditation on balance. Feel the warmth rising from the broth, listen to the bubbling simmer, and savour the calming aroma. When you eat, do so slowly acknowledging the care in each ingredient and the tradition in each bite. Kitsune Udon is humble yet deeply comforting—a quiet ritual of nourishment.

Itadakimasu. May this bowl warm both your belly and your spirit.

"Gochisōsama deshita" after eating (Thank you for the meal).

12. Sukiyaki (すき焼き / Hot Pot with Beef and Vegetables)
Prep time: 15 minutes

Serves 2–3

Ingredients:

- 250g (½ lb) thinly sliced beef (ribeye or sirloin)
- ½ block firm tofu, cut into cubes
- 1–2 cups napa cabbage, chopped
- 1 small bunch of shungiku (chrysanthemum greens) or substitute with spinach
- 1–2 spring onions, sliced diagonally
- 1 pack shirataki noodles (or glass noodles), rinsed
- 1–2 shiitake mushrooms, sliced
- 1 enoki mushroom cluster (optional)
- 1 tbsp neutral oil (like canola or grapeseed)

Sukiyaki Broth:

- ½ cup soy sauce
- ½ cup mirin
- ¼ cup sake (optional)
- 2 tbsp sugar
- ½ cup water or dashi (adjust to taste)

Instructions:

1. **Prepare the Ingredients:**
   - Arrange all ingredients neatly on a large plate or tray for easy access.
   - Mix the sukiyaki broth ingredients in a small bowl.

2. **Cook the Sukiyaki:**
   o Heat a wide, shallow pan or hot pot over medium heat. Add the oil.
   o Lightly sear the beef slices (just a few seconds each side), then push to the side.
   o Pour in the broth and bring to a gentle simmer.
   o Add tofu, cabbage, mushrooms, spring onion, and shirataki noodles in sections—don't stir. Let the ingredients slowly cook in the broth.
3. **Serve:**
   o Traditionally, sukiyaki is eaten by dipping each cooked bite into a raw beaten egg (optional), but it's delicious without too.
   o Replenish ingredients and broth as you eat. Enjoy slowly, savouring each bite.

Wellness Tip:

Sukiyaki is rich in nutrients from a variety of vegetables, mushrooms, and lean protein. By including a mix of textures and plant-based ingredients, it supports gut health and provides a satisfying, low-glycemic meal that keeps you full longer.

Mindfulness Tip:

Sukiyaki is best enjoyed as a slow, interactive meal. Be present with each step, from arranging the ingredients with care to savouring each bite. Let the rising steam, bubbling broth, and shared experience guide you into a moment of connection with your food, yourself, and others around the table.

Itadakimasu. Let this dish nourish not just your body, but your spirit.

"Gochisōsama deshita" after eating (Thank you for the meal).

13. **Shabu-Shabu (しゃぶしゃぶ / Japanese Hot Pot)**

Prep time: 20 minutes

Serves 2

Ingredients

For the broth:

- 4 cups kombu dashi (or water with a piece of kombu seaweed)
- Optional: a few slices of ginger for added warmth and flavour

For dipping:

- Ponzu sauce (citrus soy sauce)
- Sesame sauce (goma dare)

Proteins & Vegetables (thinly sliced):

- 200g beef sirloin or ribeye (shabu-shabu style thin slices)
- ½ block tofu (cut into cubes)
- 1 cup napa cabbage (chopped)
- 1 cup spinach or shungiku (edible chrysanthemum leaves)
- 1 carrot (thinly sliced)
- ½ onion (sliced)
- 1 pack enoki or shiitake mushrooms
- ½ leek or green onion (diagonally sliced)
- 1 cup cooked udon or rice for serving

Instructions

1. **Prepare the broth:**
   Heat kombu dashi in a wide pot or donabe over medium heat. Do not let it boil — remove the kombu just before boiling.
2. **Set the table:**
   Place the pot on a portable stove at the dining table. Arrange the meat and vegetables on serving plates. Set out small bowls of dipping sauces for each person.
3. **Start cooking at the table:**
   Let each person cook their own ingredients by swishing them in the hot broth ("shabu-shabu" mimics the sound of swishing!). Beef takes just a few seconds; vegetables slightly longer.
4. **Dip and enjoy:**
   After cooking, dip each item into your sauce of choice and enjoy with rice or udon.

Wellness Tip:

Shabu-shabu is naturally low in fat and high in vitamins, especially when packed with seasonal vegetables and lean protein. Using kombu dashi adds umami without salt, and the light cooking method helps preserve nutrients. It's a heart-healthy, satisfying way to eat mindfully and cleanly.

Mindfulness Tip:

Let shabu-shabu be a *slow meal*. Focus on the rhythm of cooking and eating. Swish the meat gently, notice the aroma, listen to the bubbling broth, and truly savour each bite. Invite presence at the table by pausing before and after the meal to say:

Itadakimasu. Let this dish nourish not just your body, but your spirit.

"Gochisōsama deshita" after eating (Thank you for the meal).

14. Zaru Soba (ざるそば / Cold Buckwheat Noodles)
Prep time: 15 minutes

Serves 2

Ingredients

For the soba:

- 200g soba noodles (buckwheat noodles)
- 4 cups cold water (for rinsing)
- Ice cubes (optional)

For the dipping sauce (Tsuyu):

- ¼ cup soy sauce (low sodium if preferred)
- ¼ cup mirin (sweet rice wine)
- ½ cup dashi (kombu or bonito-based broth)
- 1 tsp sugar (optional)(I never use it, but some like it)
- 1 small pinch of salt

Toppings (optional, as desired):

- 1 tsp grated daikon radish
- 1 tsp chopped green onions (scallions)
- 1 tsp toasted sesame seeds
- Wasabi (optional)
- Nori (seaweed) strips

Instructions

1. **Cook the soba noodles:**
   o Bring a large pot of water to a boil.
   o Add soba noodles and cook according to package instructions (typically 4-6 minutes). Be sure to stir gently to avoid sticking.
   o Once cooked, drain the noodles and rinse them under cold running water to remove excess starch. For a chilled version, transfer noodles to a bowl of ice water to cool completely.

2. **Prepare the dipping sauce (Tsuyu):**
   o In a small saucepan, combine soy sauce, mirin, dashi, and sugar (if using). Heat over medium heat and bring to a boil, then reduce to a simmer for 1-2 minutes. Set aside to cool.

3. **Serve the soba:**
   o Drain the noodles and serve them on a flat bamboo mat or a plate (this is what makes it "zaru soba").
   o Pour the dipping sauce into small individual bowls for each person.
   o Garnish the soba with grated daikon, green onions, sesame seeds, and nori strips if desired.

4. **Enjoy:**
   o To eat, dip the soba noodles into the dipping sauce before each bite and enjoy!

Wellness Tip:

Soba noodles, made from buckwheat, are a rich source of protein, fibre, and antioxidants, making them a fantastic choice for heart health. They are also lower in glycemic index compared to regular wheat noodles, helping to maintain balanced blood sugar levels. Paired with the light yet flavourful dipping sauce, Zaru Soba offers a refreshing and nourishing meal that's both satisfying and energizing.

Mindfulness Tip:

Eating Zaru Soba can be a calming and mindful practice. As you prepare and serve the dish, take a moment to appreciate the simple, beautiful ingredients that create the dish. When eating, focus on the sensation of each bite— the texture of the cold noodles, the umami flavour of the dipping sauce, and the balance of toppings. Pay attention to the act of dipping and savour the coolness of the soba in your mouth. It's a mindful experience that helps you slow down and be present.

Enjoy this simple, nourishing dish that offers both flavour and mindfulness with every bite!

Itadakimasu. Let this dish nourish not just your body, but your spirit.

"Gochisōsama deshita" after eating (Thank you for the meal).

15. Nikujaga (肉じゃが / Meat and Potato Stew)
Prep time: 20 minutes

Serves 2-3

Ingredients

- 200g thinly sliced beef (preferably sirloin or ribeye)
- 2 medium potatoes, peeled and cut into thin wedges or rounds
- 1 medium onion, thinly sliced
- 1 carrot, sliced into rounds (optional)
- 2 tbsp soy sauce (low sodium if preferred)
- 2 tbsp mirin (sweet rice wine)
- 1 tbsp sugar
- 1 cup dashi (kombu or bonito-based broth)
- 1 tbsp vegetable oil
- Salt and pepper to taste
- 1-2 green onions (scallions), chopped (optional, for garnish)

Instructions

1. **Prepare the ingredients:**
   - Peel and cut the potatoes into wedges or rounds.
   - Slice the onion and carrot (if using) into thin rounds.
   - Slice the beef into thin strips if it isn't already cut.
2. **Cook the beef:**
   - Heat the vegetable oil in a large pot over medium heat.

- Add the beef slices to the pot and stir-fry for about 2-3 minutes until the beef is browned. Remove the beef from the pot and set it aside.
3. **Cook the vegetables:**
   - In the same pot, add the sliced onions and carrots (if using). Stir-fry for 2-3 minutes until they begin to soften.
   - Add the potatoes to the pot and stir to combine with the onions and carrots.
4. **Simmer the dish:**
   - Return the beef to the pot and pour in the dashi, soy sauce, mirin, and sugar. Stir well to combine.
   - Bring the mixture to a boil, then reduce the heat to a simmer. Cover and cook for about 20-25 minutes or until the potatoes are tender and the flavours have melded together.
   - Season with salt and pepper to taste.
5. **Serve:**
   - Once the potatoes are cooked and the sauce has thickened slightly, remove from heat. Serve the Nikujaga in bowls and garnish with chopped green onions, if desired.

Wellness Tip:

Nikujaga combines protein-rich beef with fibre-packed potatoes and nutrient-dense vegetables, making it a well-rounded and satisfying dish. The dashi broth provides a comforting umami flavour without the need for excess salt. The balance of healthy carbs, proteins, and vegetables helps fuel the body and maintain energy levels throughout the day. The presence of mirin, a natural sweetener, adds depth to the dish without refined sugar, making it a healthier option for a hearty meal.

Mindfulness Tip:

Preparing **Nikujaga** can be an opportunity to practice mindfulness. As you slice the vegetables, focus on the texture, colour, and the motion of your knife as it moves through the ingredients. When cooking, pay attention to the smells wafting from the pot the earthy aroma of potatoes, the savoury scent of beef, and the delicate fragrance of the soy sauce and mirin. As you eat, savour each bite slowly, appreciating the combination of flavours and the nourishment it provides. Let each bite ground you in the present moment.

This easy **Nikujaga** recipe not only delivers nourishment but also offers a mindful cooking experience, allowing you to slow down, savour, and connect with the simple yet powerful act of cooking. Enjoy the comfort of this Japanese classic!

Itadakimasu. Let this dish nourish not just your body, but your spirit.

"Gochisōsama deshita" after eating (Thank you for the meal).

16. Hijiki no Nimono ひじきの煮物 (Simmered Hijiki Seaweed)

Prep time: 15 minutes

Serves 3-4 people (you need a little as a side dish)

Ingredients:

- 1/4 cup dried hijiki seaweed
- 1/2 cup sliced carrots
- 1/2 cup cooked and sliced shiitake mushrooms (or any mushrooms you prefer)
- 1/2 cup firm tofu, cubed
- 2 tablespoons soy sauce
- 1 tablespoon mirin
- 1 cup dashi (or vegetable broth for a vegetarian version)
- 1 tablespoon sesame oil
- 1 tablespoon sesame seeds (optional for garnish)

Instructions:

1. **Prepare the hijiki**: Rinse the dried hijiki seaweed under cold water to remove any impurities, then soak it in a bowl of water for about 10 minutes. Drain and set aside.
2. **Prepare the vegetables**: Slice the carrots into thin matchsticks or small rounds. If using shiitake mushrooms, slice them thinly as well.
3. **Cook the tofu**: In a pan, heat a little sesame oil and sauté the tofu cubes until golden brown on all sides. Set them aside.

4. **Simmer the dish**: In the same pan, add the remaining sesame oil. Add the carrots and shiitake mushrooms, cooking for a few minutes until softened. Then, add the soaked hijiki and stir to combine.
5. **Add liquids**: Pour in the dashi, soy sauce, mirin. Stir everything together, bring to a simmer, and cook for about 15-20 minutes until the liquid reduces slightly and the flavours meld.
6. **Finish the dish**: Gently stir in the tofu cubes and let them warm through. Serve garnished with sesame seeds if desired.

Wellness Tip:

Hijiki is a type of seaweed packed with minerals, especially calcium, iron, and magnesium, which are great for bone and muscle health. It also provides fibre, which supports digestion and helps regulate blood sugar levels. Including hijiki in your meals can enhance your overall nutrition and contribute to long-term wellness.

Mindfulness Tip:

As you prepare Hijiki, take a moment to appreciate the ingredients you're working with—each one brings a unique flavour, texture, and nutritional benefit to the dish. While cooking, breathe deeply and savour the process. Let the simmering sounds and fragrant aromas draw you into the present moment. This simple act of focusing on the task at hand can help cultivate a peaceful, meditative mindset, making your meal even more nourishing for the soul.

Itadakimasu. Let this dish nourish not just your body, but your spirit.

"Gochisōsama deshita" after eating (Thank you for the meal).

17. Kabocha no Nimono かぼちゃの煮物 (Simmered Kabocha Squash)

Prep time: 20 minutes

Serves 4 (as a side dish)

Ingredients:

- 1/2 small kabocha squash (Japanese pumpkin)
- 2 tablespoons soy sauce
- 1 tablespoon mirin
- 1 cup dashi (or vegetable broth for a vegetarian version)
- 1 tablespoon sesame oil (optional, for extra flavour)
- 1 tablespoon sake (optional, adds depth of flavour)
- 1-2 tablespoons sesame seeds (optional for garnish)

Instructions:

1. **Prepare the kabocha**: Cut the kabocha squash in half, remove the seeds, and then slice it into bite-sized wedges. There's no need to peel the kabocha as the skin is tender and adds flavour and texture to the dish.
2. **Prepare the broth**: In a medium-sized pot, combine the dashi, soy sauce, mirin, sugar, and sake (if using). Bring the mixture to a gentle simmer over medium heat.
3. **Simmer the squash**: Add the kabocha wedges to the pot and bring the mixture back to a simmer. Reduce the heat to low and cover the pot. Let the kabocha simmer for about 20-25 minutes, or until the squash is tender and the flavours are absorbed. Occasionally check to

ensure the squash is not drying out; you can add more dashi or water if needed.

4. **Finish the dish**: Once the kabocha is tender, turn off the heat and let it sit in the broth for a few minutes to further absorb the flavours. Serve the kabocha in bowls and drizzle with the remaining sauce. Garnish with sesame seeds for an added touch.

Wellness Tip:

Kabocha squash is packed with vitamins A and C, which are essential for skin health and immune function. It also contains antioxidants like beta-carotene, which support eye health and reduce inflammation. Kabocha is also a good source of fibre, which helps with digestion and supports heart health. This dish is a comforting way to nourish your body with nutrient-dense, seasonal ingredients.

Mindfulness Tip:

As you simmer the kabocha squash, take a moment to embrace the process of cooking as an act of care and presence. Notice the vibrant orange colour of the squash and the aroma of the broth as it gently simmers. When you serve the dish, be mindful of the textures and flavours that you've brought together, each ingredient plays its part in nourishing your body and soul. Allow yourself to slow down and fully experience the beauty of this meal. Let the process of cooking and eating bring you into the present moment, fostering a sense of gratitude for the food you are about to enjoy.

Itadakimasu. Let this dish nourish not just your body, but your spirit.

"Gochisōsama deshita" after eating (Thank you for the meal).

18. **Daikon no Salad** 大根のサラダ **(Daikon Radish Salad)**
Prep time 15 minutes

Serves 2 (as a side dish)

Ingredients:

- 1 medium daikon radish
- 1 tablespoon rice vinegar
- 1 teaspoon soy sauce
- 1 teaspoon sesame oil
- 1 teaspoon honey or maple syrup (optional for sweetness)
- 1 tablespoon sesame seeds (for garnish)
- 1 small carrot (optional, for colour and sweetness)
- A handful of fresh cilantro or parsley (optional, for garnish)

Instructions:

1. **Prepare the daikon**: Peel the daikon radish and slice it into thin matchstick-sized strips or use a mandolin slicer for even, thin slices. If you prefer a softer texture, you can also julienne it into slightly thicker pieces.
2. **Prepare the carrot**: If using, peel the carrot and cut it into thin matchsticks, similar in size to the daikon slices, to add colour and a touch of sweetness.
3. **Make the dressing**: In a small bowl, combine the rice vinegar, soy sauce, sesame oil, and honey or maple syrup (if using). Stir to combine and taste the dressing. Adjust sweetness or acidity to your liking.

4. **Toss the salad**: In a mixing bowl, combine the daikon, carrot, and any other optional ingredients. Drizzle the dressing over the vegetables and toss gently to coat.
5. **Garnish and serve**: Sprinkle sesame seeds over the salad for a bit of crunch and garnish with fresh cilantro or parsley if desired. Let the salad sit for a few minutes for the flavours to meld together before serving.

Wellness Tip:

Daikon radish is known for its digestive benefits. It's a natural detoxifier and helps to stimulate digestion, easing bloating and supporting a healthy gut. The high-water content in daikon also keeps the body hydrated, while the fibre aids in digestion and promotes regularity. This fresh and light salad is a great way to support your digestive health and enjoy a nutrient-packed side dish that's rich in vitamin C, antioxidants, and minerals.

Mindfulness Tip:

As you prepare this refreshing salad, focus on the textures of the daikon as you slice it—its crispness, its juiciness, and how it effortlessly glides under the blade. As you mix the ingredients together, take a moment to appreciate the colours, the aroma of the sesame oil, and the simplicity of the dish. When you sit down to enjoy the salad, savour each bite slowly, allowing the light, refreshing flavours to cleanse your palate and nourish your body. Eating with mindfulness encourages gratitude for the nourishing process and allows you to be fully present in the moment.

Itadakimasu. Let this dish nourish not just your body, but your spirit.

19. Goma-ae 胡麻和え (Sesame Spinach Salad)
Prep time: 10 minutes

Serves 2 (as a side dish)

Ingredients:

- 1 bunch of fresh spinach (about 200g)
- 2 tablespoons toasted sesame seeds (black or white)
- 1 tablespoon soy sauce
- 1 tablespoon rice vinegar
- 1 teaspoon sesame oil
- 1 teaspoon grated ginger (optional)
- 1 tablespoon sesame paste (optional, for extra richness)

Instructions:

1. **Blanch the spinach**: Bring a pot of water to a boil. Add the spinach and blanch it for about 30 seconds, until it wilts. Immediately transfer the spinach to a bowl of ice water to stop the cooking process. Drain and squeeze out excess water from the spinach. Set aside.
2. **Prepare the sesame dressing**: In a small bowl, combine the soy sauce, rice vinegar, sesame oil. If you'd like extra richness, add sesame paste and grated ginger to enhance the flavour. Whisk well to combine the dressing.
3. **Toast the sesame seeds**: In a dry skillet over low-medium heat, toast the sesame seeds for 2-3 minutes until they are lightly browned and aromatic. Be sure to stir constantly to prevent burning.

4. **Assemble the salad**: In a large bowl, chop the spinach into bite-sized pieces. Pour the dressing over the spinach and toss to coat evenly.
5. **Garnish and serve**: Sprinkle the toasted sesame seeds over the spinach and toss one more time. Serve immediately as a light and refreshing side dish or as a complement to your main meal.

Wellness Tip:

This sesame spinach salad is packed with nutrients that support your overall well-being. Spinach is a great source of iron, vitamins A, C, and K, and is rich in antioxidants. Sesame seeds, which are high in healthy fats, calcium, and magnesium, promote heart health, support bone strength, and provide a natural energy boost. The combination of these ingredients promotes a healthy immune system, glowing skin, and improved digestion.

Adding sesame paste brings an extra layer of healthy fats and a creamy texture, making the salad not only nourishing but also satisfying for a balanced diet.

Mindfulness Tip:

As you prepare this simple yet wholesome dish, focus on the textures and the colours of the ingredients. Notice the vibrant green of the spinach, the warmth of the sesame oil, and the subtle crackling sound of the sesame seeds as they toast. As you mix the spinach with the dressing, take a moment to breathe deeply and fully engage with the process. The act of cooking can be meditative—each step in preparing this dish can be a practice of mindfulness. When you sit down to enjoy your meal, be present with each bite, savouring the nutty, umami flavours and the natural sweetness of the spinach. Let each mouthful remind you to slow down and appreciate the nourishment that food brings to your body and spirit.

Itadakimasu. Let this dish nourish not just your body, but your spirit.

"Gochisōsama deshita" after eating (Thank you for the meal).

20. Shiraae 白和え (Tofu and Sesame Salad)
Prep time: 15 minutes

Serves 2-3

Ingredients:

- 200g firm tofu
- 2 tablespoons white sesame seeds (or black for a stronger flavour)
- 1 tablespoon soy sauce (or tamari for gluten-free)
- 1 tablespoon rice vinegar
- 1 teaspoon sesame oil
- 1 teaspoon mirin (optional)
- 1 tablespoon finely chopped green onions (optional for garnish)

Instructions:

1. **Prepare the tofu**: Drain the tofu and wrap it in a clean kitchen towel or paper towels. Gently press to remove excess water, then cut it into cubes or crumble it using your hands, depending on your texture preference.
2. **Toast the sesame seeds**: Place the sesame seeds in a dry skillet over medium heat. Toast them, stirring occasionally, for 2-3 minutes, until they turn golden brown and aromatic. Be sure to keep an eye on them to prevent burning. Set aside to cool.
3. **Make the sesame dressing**: In a small bowl, combine the toasted sesame seeds, soy sauce, rice vinegar, sesame oil, mirin (if using). Use a pestle or the back of

a spoon to grind the sesame seeds slightly in the bowl to release their oils and create a paste-like consistency. Stir to mix well.

4. **Assemble the dish**: In a larger bowl, gently combine the crumbled tofu or tofu cubes with the sesame dressing. Toss carefully to coat the tofu evenly in the sesame mixture.

5. **Garnish and serve**: Optionally, sprinkle finely chopped green onions over the dish for an added burst of freshness. Serve as a side dish, a light appetizer, or a healthy salad.

Wellness Tip:

Shiraae is packed with nutrients that nourish the body. Tofu is a fantastic source of plant-based protein, calcium, and iron, making it an excellent choice for bone health and muscle repair. Sesame seeds, which are rich in healthy fats, fibre, and antioxidants, promote heart health, improve skin elasticity, and support digestion. The combination of tofu and sesame seeds in Shiraae creates a well-balanced dish that aids in maintaining a healthy weight, enhancing energy levels, and supporting skin vitality. The healthy fats from sesame oil and seeds also contribute to glowing skin and improved brain function.

Mindfulness Tip:

When preparing Shiraae, take the time to notice each element in the recipe: the texture of the tofu, the warmth of the sesame oil, the aroma of the toasting sesame seeds, and the earthy flavour as you mix everything together. Be present with each step, paying attention to the rhythm of the cooking process. As you savour the dish, chew slowly and mindfully. With each bite, focus on the nutty flavour of the sesame and the soft texture of the tofu. Let the simplicity of the dish remind you of the joy in small moments and allow your senses to fully experience the nourishment you're giving your body.

Itadakimasu. Let this dish nourish not just your body, but your spirit.

"Gochisōsama deshita" after eating (Thank you for the meal).

Journal prompts for *Nourishing Our Bodies with Delicious Japanese Food*:

1. **Reflect on Your Current Diet:**
   o What are the core foods you eat on a regular basis?
   o How do they compare to the traditional Japanese foods mentioned in this chapter?
   o What are some areas where you could introduce more variety, especially fresh fruits and vegetables?
2. **Exploring Water and Tea Consumption:**
   o How much water do you drink daily?
   o Do you incorporate any teas into your daily routine? If so, which ones? If not, how might you start adding green tea or herbal teas to your day?
   o How do you feel after drinking a cup of green tea or water compared to sugary drinks?

3. **Mindful Eating and Hara Hachi Bu:**
   - What does "Hara Hachi Bu" (eating until 80% full) mean to you?
   - Do you often eat until you feel "stuffed"? How might you change this pattern?
   - Can you recall a time when you ate mindfully and felt the benefits afterward? How did it feel?

4. **The Importance of Fresh, Seasonal Foods:**
   - How often do you consume seasonal produce?
   - In what ways do you think eating seasonally might improve your health and your connection to the environment?
   - What are some seasonal fruits or vegetables that you enjoy and could start adding to your meals more regularly?

5. **Reducing Dairy and Processed Foods:**
   - How do you feel about reducing dairy or processed foods from your diet?
   - Have you ever tried plant-based milks or dairy alternatives? If so, which ones do you enjoy?
   - What are some strategies you could use to replace processed foods with fresh, whole ingredients in your daily meals?

6. **Fish and Omega-3s:**
   - How often do you consume fish, or do you have other sources of omega-3 fatty acids in your diet?
   - Are you interested in adding more fish to your meals, and if so, what types of fish would you start with?
   - How might incorporating fish or omega-3-rich foods impact your health?

7. **Cutting Down on Sugar and Additives:**
   o What are your biggest sources of sugar or artificial sweeteners in your diet?
   o How could you replace sugary snacks or beverages with healthier alternatives?
   o Have you ever tried making your own treats or snacks? What would you like to experiment with making at home?
8. **Alkalizing Foods:**
   o Are you familiar with the concept of an "alkalizing diet"? How do you feel about eating more fruits and vegetables to help balance your body's pH?
   o What alkalizing foods could you add to your daily meals, and how might you experiment with them?
   o How do you feel after eating a meal high in alkaline-forming foods?
9. **The Role of Food Presentation in Mindful Eating:**
   o How does the presentation of food influence your experience of eating?
   o Do you take time to make your meals aesthetically pleasing? How might you experiment with this?
   o What role does mindfulness play in your meals? How can you slow down to savour and appreciate the flavours and textures?
10. **Traditional Japanese Herbal Remedies:**

- Are there any herbal remedies or teas that you incorporate into your wellness routine?
- How might you explore the world of Japanese herbs and teas like **hojicha** or **matcha** for their health benefits?

- Have you noticed any positive changes in your health from consuming herbal remedies or traditional foods?

Use these prompts to reflect on your relationship with food, your health, and your connection to the principles found in Japanese food culture. Take time to explore the changes you'd like to make, and set small, achievable goals that align with a more nourishing and mindful approach to eating.

Resources:

Here is a list of Japanese books that I've read, enjoyed and took inspiration from that explore wellness rituals and concepts, offering insights into the practices and philosophies that contribute to a balanced and fulfilling life:

1. **"Ikigai: The Japanese Secret to a Long and Happy Life" by Hector Garcia and Francesc Miralles**
2. **"The Art of Simple Living: 100 Daily Practices from a Japanese Zen Monk for a Lifetime of Calm and Joy" by Shunmyo Masuno**
3. **"Wabi Sabi: Japanese Wisdom for a Perfectly Imperfect Life" by Beth Kempton**
4. **"The Book of Tea" by Kakuzo Okakura**
5. **"The Little Book of Ikigai: The Essential Japanese Way to Finding Your Purpose in Life" by Ken Mogi**
6. **"Kintsugi Wellness: The Japanese Art of Nourishing Mind, Body, and Spirit" by Candice Kumai**
7. **"The Japanese Art of Reiki: A Practical Guide to Self-Healing" by Bronwen and Frans Stiene**

8. "Kaizen: The Japanese Method for Transforming Habits, One Small Step at a Time" by Sarah Harvey
9. "The Art of Ikigai: Discovering Your Life's Purpose and Finding Happiness" by Ken Mogi
10. "Shodo: The Quiet Art of Japanese Zen Calligraphy" by Shozo Sato
11. "The Ikigai Journey: A Practical Guide to Finding Happiness and Purpose the Japanese Way" by Hector Garcia and Francesc Miralles
12. "The Art of Kintsugi: Learning the Japanese Craft of Beautiful Repair" by Alexandra Kitty
13. "The Zen of Japanese National Character: Understanding the Japanese Way of Life" by Boye Lafayette De Mente
14. "The Art of Japanese Living: Bringing Mindfulness, Joy, and Simplicity into Your Life" by Jo Peters
15. "The Japanese Art of Decluttering and Organizing" by Marie Kondo
16. "The Art of Mindful Living: Cultivating Peace and Joy in a Busy World" by Thich Nhat Hanh
17. "The Way of Tea: Reflections on a Life with Tea" by Aaron Fisher
18. "The Art of Japanese Joinery" by Kiyosi Seike
19. "The Essence of Shinto: Japan's Spiritual Heart" by Motohisa Yamakage
20. "The Art of Zen: A Way of Life in Zen Buddhism" by Stephen Addiss

These books provide a rich tapestry of insights into Japanese wellness rituals, offering guidance on how to incorporate these practices into your own life for enhanced well-being and fulfilment.

Get in touch with Barbara
www.barbaracox.me
www.barbaralovesy.com

Instagram @barbaracoxlovesy
LinkedIn – Barbara Cox Lovesy

Arigato to my Dear Family,

I am deeply grateful for your unwavering support and love, which has been a source of inspiration throughout my journey. All of your encouragement has been instrumental in bringing this book to life, and I hope it serves as a cherished guide to keep our shared legacy alive for generations to come.

As I write this, my youngest daughter Hannah, who was born in Japan in the year 2000, has just summited Mount Fuji as she has again returned to Japan for a 1-year homestay and work experience. She and her sister Lily, also born in Nara, have such deep understanding of these principles, as they grew up with them even in our daily life when we moved back to the UK.

A special thank you to my brother, Paul Saberton, for his incredible vision and talent in creating the artwork and cover for this book. Growing up surrounded by your creativity has been a true blessing and inspiring to see.

To my Dad and Mum, I am so fortunate to have each of you by my side. Dad you have always been my number 1 supporter and my dear Mum, who is with me in spirit, and her love for Japan is always remembered.

With all my love and appreciation,
Barbara x

Disclaimer

The information provided in this book is intended for educational and informational purposes only. It is not a substitute for professional advice or treatment. The author and publisher are not responsible for any actions taken based on the contents of this book. Always seek the advice of a qualified professional with any questions you may have regarding a medical condition, psychological concern, or financial situation. The author and publisher disclaim any liability for any direct, indirect, incidental, or consequential damages arising from the use of the material in this book. Your use of the information contained herein is at your own risk.

About the author

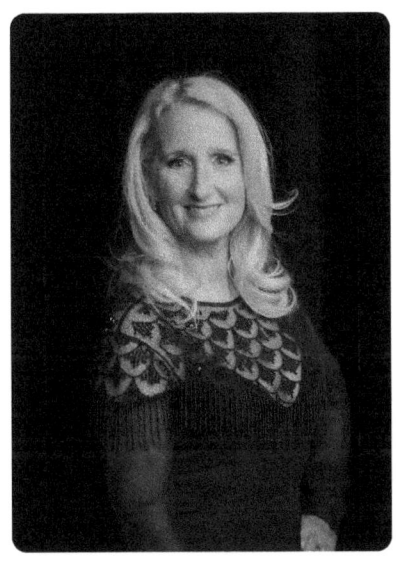

Barbara Lovesy is an award-winning renowned nutritionist, naturopath, author, and businesswoman, deeply passionate about healthy eating.

Barbara passion for the Japanese rituals of longevity blossomed during her ten-year residence in Japan, where she immersed herself in the daily practices that contribute to the country's renowned health and longevity. She observed firsthand the cultural emphasis on balanced nutrition, mindful eating, and active lifestyles, which are integral to the Japanese way of life. The tradition of incorporating nutrient-rich foods like fish, seaweed, and vegetables, along with practices such as regular physical activity and stress-reducing rituals like tea ceremonies, deeply influenced her understanding of holistic wellness. These experiences not only shaped her personal health philosophy but also inspired her professional endeavours, as she sought to integrate these principles into her work, encouraging others to embrace a lifestyle that fosters long-term health and vitality.

Beyond her professional achievements, Barbara is an Ambassador for the Cancer Active charity where you can find her first cookbook, Rainbow Recipes. In her personal life, she enjoys family time with her husband, Paul, and their four children. Together, they cherish travel, beach walks, and fossil hunting near their home on the Jurassic Coast.